Nancy Kohner is an established writer on health and social issues, and a consultant to the UK Stillbirth and Neonatal Death Society (SANDS), working with them over many years. She is the author of the Health Education Authority's original *Pregnancy Book* and *Birth to Five*. She has been programme adviser for a number of BBC television programmes — including *Having a Baby* for which she wrote the bestselling book of the same title. She was the consultant for Jonathan Miller's series *Who Cares?* and her book *Caring at Home* was requested by over 30,000 viewers. Most recently she has advised on the second series, *Who Cares Now?*, and co-written (with Penny Mares) a book to accompany it.

Alix Henley is a freelance writer, researcher and consultant. She specialises in matters to do with health and health care, and has a particular interest in communication between professionals and consumers, and in equal opportunity issues. Most recently she co-wrote, with Nancy Kohner, *Miscarriage, Stillbirth and Neonatal Death: Guidelines for Professionals* for the UK Stillbirth and Neonatal Death Society. Her other publications include *Good Practice in Hospital Care for Dying Patients*, published by the King's Fund, and, as co-author, *Health Care in Multiracial Britain*, published by the National Extension College.

# WHEN A BABY DIES

## The Experience of Late Miscarriage, Stillbirth and Neonatal Death

*Nancy Kohner and Alix Henley*

Pandora
*An Imprint of* HarperCollins*Publishers*

Pandora Press
An Imprint of HarperCollins*Publishers*
77–85 Fulham Palace Road,
Hammersmith, London W6 8JB

Published by Pandora Press 1991
10  9  8  7  6  5  4  3

© Nancy Kohner & Alix Henley 1991

Nancy Kohner and Alix Henley assert their moral right to
be identified as the authors of this work

A catalogue record for this book
is available from the British Library

ISBN 0 04 440566 9

Typeset by Harper Phototypesetters Limited,
Northampton, England
Printed in Great Britain by
HarperCollinsManufacturing Glasgow

# Contents

# Acknowledgements

We owe a great debt to the very many parents who, in different ways, have contributed to this book. We would like to thank them all, not only those who have kindly allowed us to quote from their letters, accounts or interviews, but equally those whose experiences have informed the book even though they are not quoted. Throughout the writing of the book, parents have been extraordinarily and unfailingly generous in sharing their thoughts and experiences with us, and have given us a great deal of support and encouragement.

We should also like to thank everyone at the Stillbirth and Neonatal Death Society, particularly Roma Iskander for her encouragement and her confidence in the project, Alison Melville for her practical help and hard work, Lesley Corner for stepping in so efficiently when Alison left, and Averil Rodd for sharing her understanding and expertise.

Many people contributed to and commented on the medical sections of the book and we are most grateful to all of them. In particular, we would like to thank Gaye Henson, Consultant Obstetrician at the Whittington Hospital, London, Keith Dodd, Consultant Paediatrician, Derbyshire Children's Hospital, Sandy Calvert, Consultant Neonatalogist, St George's Hospital, London, and Kevin Gangar, Lecturer in Obstetrics and Gynaecology, St Mary's Hospital, London. They have all been tremendously generous with their time and patience.

Sallie Burrows-Smith, Gill Mallinson, Judy Priest and Judith Schott have all read, commented and discussed the book with us as it progressed, and their help has been invaluable. We would also like to thank Tim Kirby for reading the book in its final draft.

Finally, we must thank several important people who have made it practically possible for us to write the book: Fred

Adelmann, Tom McGing, Lotti Henley, Tana Maclaine, Alison
Leftwich, Brenda Delany and Kim Clancy.

# Introduction

'All those hopes, all that happiness and expectation, brought to an end for no reason.'

The death of a baby, whether at birth or in the weeks or months immediately afterwards, is no less a death than any other. It is no less significant, no less important, no less heartbreaking than the death of an older child or an adult. It is certainly different, but it is not a lesser event.

The loss of a baby is the loss of a person. All parents who are positive about their pregnancy include their baby not just in their plans for the future but in their present lives too, so that even before birth, a baby begins to be considered, loved and cared for. A baby's death is also the death of a person *who would have been.* It means the ending of dreams and hopes and plans, the loss of a future. Even a baby lost in the earliest stages of pregnancy may have this significance for the parents. Parents may also have invested so much of themselves in their baby that when the baby dies, a part of them dies too. Parents who lose their first baby lose their new identity as parents; those who already have children lose an expected new member of their family.

The significance of a baby's death has not been recognised in the past and bereaved parents have often struggled alone with a grief which others have neither understood nor acknowledged. Even now, when there is better understanding of this particularly difficult kind of bereavement and when professional practice has greatly improved, one of the most common themes mentioned by parents is still their feeling of isolation.

Reading about other people's experiences can help parents to understand and make sense of what they are going through, and can give them the support of knowing that other people have been through the same or similar experiences. We hope that this book will help parents in this way. We hope too that the book will help those who care for bereaved parents to understand more about parents' experiences and needs around the time of their baby's death, and so to feel more confident about providing a service which can meet those needs appropriately.

In this book, parents tell the story of their baby's death — what happened, how they felt, and what impact it had on them and their lives. They speak about what they did and what others did for them to help them through their loss. We also offer factual information on what is currently known about why babies die, and we look at such issues as hospital practice, professional attitudes, the nature of bereavement, the process of grieving, sources of support and future pregnancies.

We have focused on loss through late miscarriage, stillbirth and neonatal death (death within the first twenty-eight days of life). But much of what we have written, and some of the accounts we have used, are also about early miscarriage, the loss of a baby following a termination, and the loss of older babies.

The book is based on the experiences of many hundreds of parents. It uses the letters and accounts which bereaved parents have written over many years to the UK Stillbirth and Neonatal Death Society (SANDS). We have supplemented these written accounts with interviews, and have also used accounts from parents who have written to other organisations which offer support to bereaved parents. What we have written has been guided by our material: we have dealt with those things that parents have written and told us about.

Although we have not selected the accounts we have used in any scientific way, they represent a wide range of experiences and backgrounds. Many common themes recur throughout the material and it is clear that much is shared by all bereaved parents, no matter how or at what stage they have lost their baby. It is this shared experience that we have particularly wanted to record, and it is the purpose of the book to share it with others.

# 1 Parents' Stories

These are the stories of parents whose babies died, either before birth or afterwards. Their stories are not typical because there is no such thing as a typical story. For each parent, the experience of losing a baby is painfully individual. It can also be very isolating. Parents feel that what has happened to them has not happened, *cannot* have happened, to anyone else before — and in a way, they are right.

Yet almost all parents who have lost a baby will recognise in these stories something which connects with their own experience. And just as it helps some parents to write down all that happened to them and to their baby, so it helps others to read their stories.

## ANGELA'S STORY

**Angela's baby daughter, Suzanne, died twenty-eight hours after she was born. Angela wrote this account five months after Suzanne's death.**

This is the first time I've been able to put pen to paper to tell anyone how I feel about the death of my much-loved daughter, Suzanne Alicia, who was born on 11 December and who died twenty-eight hours later.

The day of her birth began with excitement and relief. Soon my child would be born and the pain I was in would soon be gone (or so I thought). I had to go into hospital to be induced because she was late, so I said goodbye to my two sons, Daniel, aged 8, and Matthew, aged 5, and said I would see them the next day with our new baby. My husband drove me to the hospital.

I was induced at 11 a.m. and Suzanne was born at 12.55 p.m., so her birth was quick and very good. She was a healthy, 8lb, beautiful girl. We couldn't believe we had a daughter to add to our sons. We were elated, and I felt I'd been given all I had ever wanted in the world. I almost felt like pinching myself to see if it was a dream.

I fed her at 5.15 but she wasn't very interested. She seemed tired and soon went back to sleep. My mum and auntie came to see her, then later my husband and a friend, Yvonne. Yvonne held her and we chatted. I mentioned that Suzanne seemed a bit blue, but I wasn't concerned. Alan (my husband) held her for about thirty minutes and she seemed to pink up, so I thought she must have been cold.

After they'd left, I had a bath and while I was in it I heard her cry. So I got out and dressed but when I got back she'd gone back to sleep. I woke her at 9.45 as she was still asleep and she needed her next feed, but she really didn't want it. The midwife brought me some expressed milk for her and she gulped an ounce of it. I talked to her and told her she'd have wind. When I tried to wind her, I felt her hair against my cheek. I kept talking and kissing her, telling her how much I loved her. Then the midwife came and took her down to the nursery. In the night I heard her screaming, as though someone was touching her and it was hurting. I felt upset, but she went quiet again.

Just past midnight, the midwife came to say she was admitting Suzanne to the special care baby unit. I was alarmed but she soon calmed me down, saying it was a precautionary measure because Suzanne was moaning and rather blue. The doctor came to see me. He was lovely and said Suzanne seemed OK but it was better to be safe than sorry. I phoned Alan and told him, but said don't worry as no one else seemed to be.

They brought Suzanne to say goodbye to me. I kissed her and said she'd be fine. Later they brought me a photo of her in the SCBU [the special care baby unit] and said she was peaceful and asleep, so I relaxed again.

At 4.45 a.m. the midwife came back and said Suzanne was worse. I rang Alan and he said he would go to the SCBU. About three hours later Alan walked through the door and as soon as I saw his face I knew it was bad. He couldn't speak for a while and just sobbed on my bed. Eventually, after frantic questioning, he told me that she had got too big a liver and spleen, and a serious chest infection, and she had already almost died twice. I couldn't believe it, I thought he'd got it wrong.

I discharged myself and we went up there. (The SCBU is in a separate hospital.) We had to wait nearly two hours in the waiting room because Suzanne was fighting for her life, but when I saw her, I couldn't believe my eyes. She was a better colour than she had been since she was born, and awake, alert and kicking. I couldn't believe that she was going to die. I felt they had to be wrong.

But by the afternoon all my hope for her recovery had gone. I can't begin to describe what it was like, watching her deteriorate the way she did. I couldn't speak to her or anyone, I just cried and willed her to live. She never opened her eyes again or moved. In the morning she had clung to my finger, but not so now, she was turning more blue and my baby was dying. She was attached to all sorts of machines and towards the end of the afternoon, I prayed she would die because her hands were black from tubes, and the ventilator was doing her breathing. At 5 o'clock my prayers were answered and my world fell apart.

We were allowed to stay with her as long as we wished. My family and friends came, cried and held her. She was bathed and dressed. She looked so beautiful it still hurts to think about it.

We left the hospital at 8.30 p.m. I felt like I wanted to run so far away from that place. The funeral took place ten days later and a post-mortem revealed that she died of pneumonia and septicaemia.

I really believe I was in shock for about three weeks, I was so calm and collected, but now is the time my pain goes on and on, I feel so desperate, so alone. All I want to do is talk, talk, talk about her. My boys are at school all day and I spend my time in her world. I keep trying to do what people say and live for my husband and family, but what do I do with all my love and my pain for Suzanne? She was my life, the daughter Alan and I had always wanted. How do I live my life knowing I had her and lost her so quickly?

## ANN'S STORY

**Ann's baby son was stillborn. At the very end of her pregnancy, Ann realised she could no longer feel her baby's**

**movements, and when she was monitored, no heartbeat could be found.**

We had been trying for a family for over two years and I was being seen by an infertility specialist when I found out I was pregnant. We were absolutely thrilled, and as this was just before Christmas, it made it a very special time.

I had a wonderful pregnancy without any trouble. I didn't suffer from any morning sickness or any of the other niggling complaints usually associated with pregnancy. I left my job in June. I was sad to leave because I really enjoyed my work, but as it was so important to me to bring up my baby myself, I didn't have any intention of going back to work afterwards. I spent the next few months at home, planning and buying absolutely everything for the baby. We decorated the room. Everybody was really excited. I did all the right things. I don't smoke and I didn't drink alcohol, and I ate well. I attended relaxation classes, bought lots of books and learnt as much as I could.

When my date of delivery was changed through hormone tests and scans, from 10 August to 26 August, it didn't alarm anybody. I'd always had a long cycle (between six to seven weeks) so the new date seemed to make more sense.

I had my last scan at about thirty-five weeks and everything was fine. A few weeks later, I was told the baby had engaged. It was just a case of waiting now. I carried on being really healthy and my friends remarked how much pregnancy seemed to suit me and how I was 'blooming'.

In the last few weeks, the baby didn't move so much and I mentioned this at my check-ups. But I was always reassured that this was normal as the baby had less room to move towards the end and as long as I was getting at least ten kicks a day, I was not to worry. I always got far more than this, so again, no one was concerned. I carried on noting my tenth movement on a kick chart and took it in with me each week.

Then on 28 August, two days after my due date, I didn't feel anything. At 6 o'clock, when my husband came home from work, I rang the hospital. The nurse said not to worry as I may be going into labour and that the baby may be in distress. She asked us to come in and be monitored for an hour or so.

We arrived at the hospital in quite good spirits, thinking that we would just be reassured that everything was fine and secretly hoping that they'd keep me in and deliver the baby! We were totally unprepared for the nightmare which followed.

After being shown into the admission room, a nurse examined me and tried to pick out the heartbeat on the monitor. After a while, she said that the machine was probably faulty and she left to get another one. When she returned with a senior nurse, I began to worry. Again the heartbeat couldn't be found. She said that sometimes babies lie in funny positions and it makes the heartbeat difficult to trace. A doctor finally arrived. By this time I was petrified. She tried in vain for what seemed like ages. Then she told us that our baby was dead.

I cannot explain the feelings inside me. Sheer desolation. And panic, knowing that I would have to give birth to a dead baby. I kept wanting to know why, why, why? I demanded a scan, desperately hoping that they would find it was some dreadful mistake. We clung to this faint hope until it was finally proved to me that my baby was dead.

I was admitted to a private room and my husband stayed with me. He stayed with me the whole time I was in hospital, twenty-four hours a day. If we hadn't been together, I don't think either of us could have coped. That night was the most frightening and devastating night of our lives. I fought off all the drugs and sleeping tablets I had been given. We just kept willing the baby to kick.

The next day I was induced and my baby was born at 2.13 a.m. He was taken away and dressed and brought back to us. We were left alone with him. He was the most beautiful baby I have ever seen. Our love for him was overwhelming. We could have held and nursed him all night. He was so perfect, a beautiful 5lb 4oz little boy who looked as if he was asleep.

When he was finally taken away, I felt such emptiness and bewilderment. Why did this happen to us?

We were told that he had died because of placental insufficiency: the placenta was too small. They said that what had probably happened was that over the last few weeks of pregnancy the placenta had deteriorated slowly so that he got less food and oxygen and got weaker and weaker, until finally he would have 'gone to sleep'. I hope he never suffered.

## KEVIN'S STORY

**Kevin's second daughter, Lara, was born by emergency caesarean. Melissa, his wife, was very ill and had to have a hysterectomy. Lara lived for fifteen hours.**

Two months on we still cannot fully believe what has happened. Melissa and I had been looking forward so much to the arrival of our second child. Boy or girl? It didn't matter: 'So long as everything is OK,' that's what I said to people.

Melissa finally went into labour twelve days late. No worries, as Kaly our first child (now 2½ years old) was eighteen days late. We phoned the hospital — just as we had done for Kaly — at 2.30 a.m. on Sunday. My mum and dad came over to look after Kaly. I saw the excitement in their eyes, knowing their second grandchild was on its way. All the waiting would soon be over. Boy or girl, it didn't matter, 'As long as everything was OK.'

We drove off in thick fog, Melissa lying in the back of the car because her contractions were strong. After a slow drive, we arrived at the hospital, all OK. In the labour suite, the baby's heart rate was strong and Melissa was progressing quickly. Everything was so similar to Kaly's birth. I remembered her being passed to me and her eyes looking at me. That moment was so precious.

Melissa had to have a drip to encourage labour as there had been no change in her dilation for three hours. But we reached the final stage. And then it all went wrong. It was a nightmare. The monitor showed the baby was in distress. Forceps were tried — but weren't successful because the head was in the wrong position. Suddenly the doctor called for an emergency caesarean. What was happening? Their faces said it all, though they were trying to reassure me.

They wheeled Melissa to the theatre and I waited in a separate room. It was then my tears began. Why was this happening to us? We had had our share of tragedy and upset in recent years. Surely they would both be all right?

Heather, the midwife, joined me. We drank tea and she cried with me. It was very hard for her too, and her support will never be forgotten. Another nurse and the sister came and talked. I still cried, mainly with disbelief. Then a nurse arrived with the news that Lara had been born at 4.20 p.m. but that it had taken twenty minutes to get a heart rate. She would have to go to the special care unit on a respirator. Her chances were very slim and she could be brain damaged.

Melissa was still in theatre. I had to see the consultant. He explained that my wife had ruptured her womb and lost four pints of blood. This had caused the baby distress. The only safe course was a hysterectomy, which was performed immediately. I can remember thinking at the time, 'There's no way Melissa will want another pregnancy.' But as the weeks have gone by, the fact that we can have no more children becomes harder and harder to come to terms with. It seems to leave a void in our lives.

I was very numb. It was like sleep-walking. I went to see Lara. As she lay in the incubator, my one overwhelming wish was to hold her. She looked so much like her sister at birth — dark hair, long fingernails. But I would never see her eyes open. I touched her. I couldn't hold her because she was all wired up.

The nurses in the SCBU were so nice, but they gave little hope. She had suffered such a lot in such a short time. It was hard to believe my daughter was in this unit with premature babies. She weighed 8lb 2oz — 2oz more than Kaly — and she was so perfect.

The hospital chaplain was introduced to me. He became a great comfort to Melissa and me. Lara was baptised and Heather, our midwife, was godparent.

Then I had to make the phone calls. I rang my mum. The words just wouldn't come out and the tears flowed. My dad came to the hospital and was allowed to see Lara. I do hope that helped him, I believe it did.

I said goodnight to Melissa and explained about Lara — that there was little hope. But Melissa was still very weak and on drugs. It wasn't fair to expect her to take it all in, and I didn't mention the hysterectomy.

I stayed with my parents that night. I hugged my mum. I remember saying this was the worst day of my life, and we both cried. I went to see Kaly, asleep in her bed. She somehow made me feel better.

On 1 May, Lara died. She lived just fifteen hours. Melissa and I both held her, took pictures and said goodbye. She was so perfect. We wish now we had spent more time with her, but at least we have some memories and they are precious to us both.

Two months on, I still wake up and think it hasn't happened and that Melissa is still expecting Lara. It hurts when people think you are 'over it' because we will never get over what happened. I remember saying in the hospital that part of us died with her.

I felt very close to Lara. I know I didn't carry her for nine months, but I wanted her so badly.

## JOAN'S STORY

**When she was seventeen weeks pregnant, Joan began to bleed. Later, in hospital, she went into labour.**

After four years of waiting to get pregnant, then having had a miscarriage at twelve weeks, I discovered that I was pregnant. I was shocked at first, but my husband John and my daughter Carla (then aged 7) were over the moon. It took me a few weeks to get used to the idea, but then I really looked forward to having a baby.

I began to suffer with all-day sickness and I took this as being a good sign. We were all very concerned until I passed the twelve-week stage, and once I did we were all very excited about the baby.

Then, at about seventeen weeks pregnant, one Wednesday afternoon, I began to get niggly pains in my side. I tried to ignore them as much as I could and carry on as normal. When we went to bed that night it was uncomfortable to lie on one side. I did go to sleep, but at about 4 a.m. I awoke with really bad pains. I got up and went to the toilet and discovered that I was bleeding. I was shocked and I froze to the spot for a few moments, then I called John. I began to shout 'Please God, no. Please God, no.' John phoned the doctor who said go back to bed and rest, and if needed she would call in the morning.

The next morning I was still bleeding. The doctor called but could not find the baby's heartbeat, so she phoned the midwife. The midwife talked to the consultant, who knew me well, and I was admitted to hospital, to the antenatal ward instead of the gynae ward. Looking back I was grateful for that because having experienced both, I felt that antenatal was geared up for having babies, not losing them, so I felt less stressed.

After being examined by the doctor and put on a fetal monitor, they still could not find a heartbeat. This made me really worried. The doctor told me that I could have a scan the next day and not to worry, but I did worry non-stop.

Later that day the pain moved around to the front, low down, and became uncomfortable. I tried to sleep but couldn't. I called the midwife a few times but I felt I was disturbing everyone. The pain became unbearable, so I got up and went out into the corridor. I kept trying to think of reasons for the pain — cramp, infection — but I suppose deep down I knew that there was something terribly wrong. The midwife gave me some pethidine and let me sleep in another room, alone. I started to bleed a lot more and began to panic. I remember thinking, no, I can't be losing my baby, I love him so much. I can't let him die. He's too small, he won't survive. Why did I get pregnant, out of the blue, just to lose him? What on earth would be the point?

After a while I went to sleep, and when I woke up in the morning, the pain had gone. Although I was still bleeding, I felt relieved. The bleeding carried on all morning and about midday I had a scan. I was really happy to see the baby move on the scan, to see his tiny heart beating. I couldn't wait to see John and Carla to tell them. Although the scan showed the placenta was low down, I kept thinking he would be all right.

Later that day the pain came back and I went into labour. After going through the worst pain and torment of my life, I most reluctantly gave birth at 12.20 a.m. to our tiny baby. I think I felt him kick my thigh. I didn't want to look in case he was still alive. I was sure he was, if only for a few seconds. I could not bear the thought of him suffering.

After a few minutes, I asked the midwife if I could see him. She told me what to expect so that I would not be shocked, and after cleaning him, she brought him in so I could see him. I was very scared at first, but when I looked at him, he was the most beautiful baby I have ever seen — apart from Carla. I loved him so much I could not cry then. I wanted to hold him but didn't ask. I felt so sad for him. Why did he have to die? I could not understand why my body had rejected him, he was so perfect. I remember looking at his tiny hands and fingers. Why couldn't those little hands have reached out for me to cuddle him? I love him so much. It hurt, it still hurts, it always will.

I asked the midwife what would happen to him. She quietly said, 'Through the normal hospital system.' I could not bear that and asked if I could take him home and bury him in the garden. She said she did not really know and would check with the doctor. The doctor said he didn't see why not, but would check with the consultant. I was then taken to the theatre, as the placenta had not detached. I remember waking up at about 4 a.m. and it really hit me then. I cried and cried.

The next morning I phoned John. He was so upset. But the hardest thing was telling Carla. They both came to the hospital as soon as they could. They were in the room with me when the consultant came in. He said it was not possible for me to bury my baby in my garden, it was against the law. But after seeing how upset I was, he did say that he would check with the administrator on Monday morning, but the baby must stay in the hospital until then.

Having to leave the hospital that day without the baby was awful. It was a really hard weekend to get through, not knowing what was going to happen to him. But on Monday morning I had a phone call from the administrator of the maternity unit, who was very understanding and kind. She said I was perfectly within my rights to bury him in my garden as long as I checked with the Environmental Health Officer. But she said I could also bury him in a little cemetery near my home — and that is what we chose to do.

On a rainy Thursday morning, our little boy was put to rest in his tiny grave. The chaplain said a lovely verse, and me, John and Carla said our goodbyes.

## HAYRIYE'S STORY

**Hayriye's second son, Serdar, was premature and suffered brain damage as a result of lack of oxygen in the womb. He lived for three months, and was always very poorly.**

My second child was born prematurely at thirty-three weeks by emergency caesarean. Nobody knows how long Serdar was in distress but he suffered from a lack of oxygen as the placenta tore and I had internal bleeding. The damage was already done in the womb. He began to fit very soon after birth.

I was told during the night that my baby was twitching and had a high-pitched cry. This was abnormal. I was shattered at this news. They said it may be the lack of oxygen in the womb and if so it would take thirty-six hours for the fits to stop. Serdar never did stop fitting. He fitted for long periods. I asked if my baby was in pain while he was fitting and crying at the same time. They said they didn't think so, but I felt he was, the way he clenched his tiny fists and pulled his knees up to his tummy. It tore me to pieces.

I was in hospital for eight days. I had an empty cot at the end of my bed that constantly made me cry. I couldn't talk to anyone without crying; I couldn't even talk, I was so choked all the time. The special care baby unit had sent me a photo of my baby and I held it to my heart and cried.

The day I left hospital was strange. As we came out of the hospital, I felt as if I was walking out into a different world. Everything had changed, even my home looked different.

I visited Serdar every day in hospital for twelve weeks. He never came home. The only way I could cope was dealing with one day at a time. If Serdar had a reasonably good day, so did I. If he had a bad day, I did too.

At three weeks old Serdar went for a head scan. They found extensive damage on the thinking part of his brain. There was a permanent lump in my throat. Whenever a doctor spoke to us I cried. I wasn't weak like everyone thought. I just had to cry and let out my grief and sadness because it was choking me. The crying helped me to be stronger, to cope with the next day and the next.

Serdar's doctor told us his outlook was very poor. She said that if you cut off a leg it won't grow back, and Serdar's brain damage was the same. I wasn't sure what this meant and asked if he'd walk or talk. She said, 'My dear, I don't expect him to survive.'

I would not give up on my baby, never. I told the doctors they were not God and could be wrong. That is what I wanted to believe. He was alive, breathing by himself — there was hope. I had tremendous hope. A sister in special care said she wasn't sure it was a good thing to have too much hope, but I don't think I could have lived through it without hope.

I made up my mind to be with Serdar as often as I could. Deep down I felt that time was short. I fed him with a bottle and a tube, bathed him, dressed him, gave him his medicine. Best of all, we had loads of cuddles. Serdar's fits were the major problem. The medical team couldn't control them as they wanted to. He used up all his energy fitting. Towards the end, his tiny body couldn't cope. He began to sweat excessively. Very soon he had become dehydrated. His eyes had sunk in, there was a hollow in his tummy and he was paler.

The day before Serdar died he was very ill and wouldn't settle at all. Previously he had stopped breathing in my arms but the nurses 'bagged' him and he began to breathe. This happened twice as I was feeding him. I knew this was a warning to me. I said to one doctor, 'One day I'll have to bury him. I can't do it, I can't put him under the ground.'

Serdar died on 8 May, a day after his brother's third birthday. The call came at 11.30 p.m. My husband had just come back from visiting Serdar half an hour before. Alone, I rushed to the hospital. My husband waited for my mum to come and stay with our other son. I was met by three nurses who tried to calm me down: 'We did all that we could, he went peacefully.' I wanted to be with him when he died, I wanted to. I was led to his cot. He was wrapped up in a little bundle. I held him close to me. 'I love him so much, so much,' I kept saying.

We were moved to a little room. As soon as I held Serdar after he'd died I felt an incredible peace, a calm, as if a storm had suddenly stopped. I felt Serdar was where he wanted to be, at peace with God. The doctor said Serdar almost had a smile on his face. I agreed. He had fought enough.

Before Serdar died, I had said to the doctor that if he died I wanted to take him home until I buried him. We are Muslims and bury our dead within a few days. He said I could. But the night sister said they don't do that. I also asked to wash my baby, but she said she must do it, it was her job. She filled a bowl of water and washed him with that hard paper towel while I cried and watched her. I feel very angry with myself. I wish I had stood up to her and demanded to wash my baby. Nobody had more right than me. My husband told her too, but she didn't allow us.

Afterwards I held Serdar again, so did his dad. They took

photos of us together. They break me up inside to see them but I'm glad I have them. I clung to my baby, not wanting to be separated from him. I didn't want him to be put in the mortuary. After several hours, the sister came to take Serdar. She said, 'Another one will come, another one will come.' I didn't want another one, I wanted Serdar.

## VAL'S STORY

**Val had twin daughters, Samantha and Kathryn. They were born prematurely. Samantha survived, but Kathryn died.**

'Are there twins in the family?' the nurse asked me as I was being scanned at ten weeks. 'No, why?' 'Because it's twins!' she announced. I looked carefully at the picture. I wanted to see this for myself. They were there all right, one not quite as clear as the other, but there they were. I couldn't believe it! But after the initial shock, I became so excited, thinking about two of everything.

I phoned Geoff, my husband. How would he take it? I couldn't wait to get home, so I phoned him from a phone box outside the hospital. 'Geoff, you'll never guess, it's twins!' No response. 'Geoff?' I heard him laughing and I knew he thought he'd done something special. Twins! Thrilled to bits — absolutely.

Take it easy, everybody kept telling me. Then, at fifteen weeks, I had a show. What, me? I'm as healthy as anything. There must be something wrong. Just take it easy, the doctor told me. How can you take it easy with a demanding toddler? I had two sets of pains lasting an hour each time at twenty and twenty-two weeks. Then at twenty-four weeks, I developed thrush, which left me with a watery, bloody discharge that just got worse and worse as the weeks went by. At twenty-seven weeks it was confirmed — my worst fear — that my membranes had ruptured.

'Stay in hospital? With a toddler to look after? You're joking.' They weren't. I had no choice. I couldn't risk any infection with my waters breaking. I had to do what was best. Complete bed rest, they said, for thirteen weeks, and no parole at weekends.

The nurses and staff at the hospital were almost my family for the ensuing weeks and undoubtedly helped me through it. Every time it seemed that the waters were sealing, I would start losing blood again. There was something definitely wrong, there had to be. The scans kept showing one baby always smaller than the other and it was very worrying. At thirty weeks I had an X-ray. The babies appeared to be the same size, but one was obviously thinner than the other. Nothing to worry about, they said, but I still worried.

Thank God for my husband. He was coping very well with Michael, our 18-month-old son, and family and friends were helping out constantly, as Geoff still had to go to work. His manager at work also helped tremendously by letting him have as much time off as he needed to relieve the pressure on him. Our families gave us all the moral support they could to get us through it. I didn't have to worry, just 'enjoy the rest while you can'. I managed to get to thirty-four weeks when suddenly I went into labour and an emergency section was hurriedly arranged.

Two little girls! Lovely! Were they all right? Yes, fine — one was 4lb 2½oz and the other was 3lb 6oz. They had gone to the special care baby unit and were both on oxygen. Nothing to worry about. Geoff brought me a blurred photograph of each of them, which the hospital routinely take. They looked OK, I thought. He also told me that the little one had to have more oxygen than the other and I told him not to 'worry me with every little thing'. I feel terrible about saying that now.

The vicar came and said they would have to be baptised, the little one was very poorly. But they tell everybody this, I thought, being a low birth weight and needing oxygen. Very poorly. I just didn't take it in at all. So what should we name them? We decided then and there on Samantha Jayne and Kathryn Ann, and they were baptised. Kathryn was the little one.

I went to see them the next morning. I saw Samantha first, not needing oxygen now. Lovely. Then Kathryn. 'You do realise she's very poorly, don't you?' Not really, no. 'Yes,' I said.

She looked squashed against a sheet in the incubator and was covered from the chest down with another sheet. I realise why, now. Nothing registered at all and I went back to my bed. I kept looking at the pictures. One of the staff I knew from antenatal came and gave me her rosary beads. I said, 'You're not trying to worry me, are you?' 'No,' she said. What else could she say? It still didn't dawn on me.

Geoff arrived with my sister and he went to see them. He came back with a terrible look on his face. He told me there were three doctors around her. I said he'd better get back to the SCBU, and he went.

At that point, all my family arrived to visit. I sent them all up to the SCBU. I said to my mum, 'Mum, she's poorly, she's not going to make it.' Mum rushed up to see her. I was alone in a ward full of people. What's happening, I thought. I was worried. It was only then that I seemed to realise all at once that she was going to die.

The nurse came with a wheelchair and told me that the doctor wanted to see me. Then I knew. I asked why, and she just told me politely to sit in the wheelchair.

The inevitable had happened. She wheeled me into a single room where Geoff was sitting with a doctor. The doctor told me that Kathryn had died. I broke down and cried. I finally realised what had been going on: 100 per cent oxygen, X-rays, pneumonia in her lung — collapsed and couldn't be ventilated — died. We were devastated. The doctor explained everything. She also explained that Kathryn had a 'squashed' appearance known as talipes. The doctor asked if we would like to hold her and we said yes.

After the family had shared our grief, they went home. We held Kathryn then. We took two pictures of her. We didn't know why we were taking them, we just knew we had to.

Geoff had to make all the arrangements for her funeral. We knew the undertakers and the vicar, so it was a very private, personal service. We bought two red roses, one from Samantha, one from Michael, and put them on her little coffin. Geoff and I wanted to go alone, so we didn't ask our families to come, and they respected our wishes. It was just something we had to do by ourselves, and they understood. We chose to have her cremated and her ashes were scattered on the garden at the crematorium.

As the funeral was only three days after I'd had the caesarean, I chose to go back to the hospital to complete my period of recuperation. The truth was I just couldn't face going home without two babies. Geoff had to go home to see to Michael, and also to see to removing the 'spare' cot from the twins' bedroom before I came home.

I came home the following weekend, just before Christmas. Geoff had made the most tremendous effort, cleaning the house and putting the decorations up. It was lovely. After being cooped up in a hospital room for seven weeks, it was like a palace. And Michael — he was so pleased I was home he didn't let me out of his sight and had a beaming smile on his face all the time.

We still had to go back to the hospital to give Samantha her breast milk and her share of love and attention, but all the time we wished she was at home. Finally, after three and a half weeks, the day came to take her home. Oh, what a terribly sad day, so sad. It should have been the happiest day in our lives, taking our twins home. Samantha we had, Kathryn we had not.

Good night, God bless, darling. We wish we could hold you now.

## SHARON'S STORY

**A routine scan during her pregnancy showed that Sharon's baby was anencephalic and would not survive. She and her husband Ian decided to end the pregnancy.**

When I was seventeen weeks pregnant, I went for my routine scan. I wasn't overly concerned as my first pregnancy had been normal enough. I had noticed that I hadn't gained much weight, and I hadn't the same enthusiasm to knit or look at baby clothes as I did with my first pregnancy, but I just put it down to second time around. (Maybe it was mother's intuition, I don't know.)

Before leaving the scan room, the doctor said she would like to see me the following week as she wasn't sure if the baby was developing properly. It was difficult during the next week, not knowing what we were going to be told. I had noticed something different about the scan, having had one for our first child.

On returning the following week, with my husband, I went in to be scanned while he waited outside. The doctor scanned and found the baby's position. She looked around for a few minutes and said, 'It's as I thought. The baby's skull hasn't formed properly. Your baby is not going to survive.' I started to cry, I just didn't know what to say. She dried up my tears and called my husband in and showed him what was wrong with the baby. The doctor had to be completely sure of her findings so she called in another doctor who confirmed the devastating news. He said that we would have to decide within forty-eight hours what we were going to do. Our choice was to continue with the pregnancy, with the chance of carrying the baby to full term and the possibility of the baby living an hour or not at all, or having the pregnancy terminated. We both left the hospital devastated. We sat in the car holding one another, just crying and crying.

We had to go and break the news to our parents and try and get ourselves in the right state of mind to make the hardest decision of our lives. I don't think we ate or slept that weekend, working everything out. Finally, we decided to go ahead with the termination, outlining certain conditions — that my mum and mum-in-law could see the scan before I had the operation, that we could see the baby, name the baby and, lastly, that we could bury the baby at a cemetery of our choice.

At first, when we asked the doctor he wasn't sure. He kept referring to the baby as a fetus, as by then I was just over nineteen weeks, but he agreed, and I went into the hospital and that afternoon our daughter, Sarah, was born. The doctor showed Ian the baby and explained exactly what was wrong with her. She was anencephalic and her spine wasn't formed properly.

The following day, I was taken in a wheelchair, with my husband, to the mortuary where Sarah lay on the table with a white cloth over her. She was so tiny. I just looked at her. I never held her, I didn't know if I was allowed. I stayed a few moments and then went back to my room.

My dad organised the funeral for the next day. We had a service in the little room beside the mortuary. My dad, Ian's dad and Ian's grandfather led the service. We had our close relations, including our little boy. Ian then put the coffin in the back of the car and took her to the nearby cemetery where she was buried with my grandmother and uncle. I went back to my room where one of the nurses prepared tea and biscuits for myself and the relations.

The staff were really wonderful. Everyone treated me really well. There was only one doctor who made a rather upsetting remark. He said, pointing to the maternity unit, 'I will see you over there next year, having a nice healthy baby.' It seemed as if he didn't care. All he was interested in was healthy babies.

## PENNY'S STORY

**During her pregnancy, Penny was told that her baby would not survive. Her son was born when she was thirty-one weeks pregnant and he lived for four days.**

I lost my baby son ten months ago. He was four days old and very sick. Everyone was very kind to me and told me 'it was for the best' (I hate that saying), and that time would ease the pain. But every day is getting harder, especially now the 'anniversaries' are here. A year ago today, when I was five months pregnant, I was given a detailed scan which revealed that my baby had heart failure and a lot of fluid in his tummy. I was kept in hospital for a week and I was monitored every three hours just to check there was still a heartbeat. The doctors told me that they were expecting my baby to die inside me.

But he didn't. I went back to the hospital for a scan every week, and each time the doctors were amazed at the way he was fighting to survive. I was given drugs to try to put the heart right and to reduce the fluid, but after nine weeks, when I was twenty-nine weeks pregnant, I was told things were getting worse and there was nothing anyone could do. I was given the option of a termination, and after discussing it with my husband, I refused. As long as our baby wanted to fight, we would fight with him.

Very kindly, the doctors told me to be prepared for my baby to be stillborn. If he was born alive, they doubted he would last an hour.

So, on Saturday 13 August, when I was thirty-one weeks pregnant, at home alone with my 18-month-old daughter, my waters broke, and I cried. I tried sitting, standing, lying down to stop it, but there was nothing I could do. When my husband came home from work four minutes (it felt like four hours) later, I went straight to the hospital.

We'd talked and decided, with the doctors' approval, that when I went into labour, we'd let nature take its course. So no monitors were used until the very last minute. After a few minutes, the nurse found a heartbeat and I gave birth to a live baby boy at 5.47 a.m. on Sunday. His face was purple with bruises because of all the water I had carried, and his stomach was very large, but to me he was the most beautiful baby ever. I held him for forty-five minutes and cried as I watched him gasping for life, until the doctor had to admit that they'd been proved wrong about him not having the strength to live. So he was taken to the neonatal unit.

When he was three days old, I plucked up courage and asked what his chances were. The doctor said he was doing extremely well, things were definitely looking up. Later that afternoon, he was put on a ventilator, although for the previous twenty-four hours he had been breathing by himself. The nurse looking after him (we called him Ryan) explained that premature babies often forget to breathe and the ventilator was so that they didn't need to prod him to remind him to breathe. He was still on the ventilator when I left him to go to bed, but nothing else seemed wrong.

Next morning, before breakfast, the doctor came and sat down on the end of my bed. I cried before he even spoke. Even now I can remember every single word. 'Baby Ryan has had a very bad night. Although we drained the fluid off his tummy, it's now returned as bad as before, we don't know why. We did a brain scan this morning which revealed a lot of bleeding on one side of his brain. He also needs 100 per cent oxygen. I'm sorry we can't save him. Do you want to see him?' What a stupid question. I went to see him. The sides of his incubator were down, his teddy bears were by his head. Every now and then he jumped — convulsions, the doctor said. My husband came in and together we held Ryan's hands until a vicar came to baptise him.

Then my husband went to fetch our daughter Kirstie, and both our parents. I sat alone in a little room while all Ryan's tubes were removed. When my husband came back, a nurse brought Ryan to us, wrapped in blankets. His mouth was still open where the ventilator had been and his left eye was still half open. Still fighting, right to the end — although the doctor didn't know if he was conscious. I held him until his eye closed, pleaded with him to breathe just one more breath, but he didn't. The doctor came back to listen to his heart but all he said was 'He's gone.'

Every night since then I've cried, with sadness and guilt and sometimes anger. I keep going over and over the months I was pregnant, trying to think of what I did wrong. I saw a psychiatrist for a few months but all he told me was to pull myself together,

I wasn't the first woman to lose a baby and I wouldn't be the last. Besides, I was only 20, I could have plenty more. But I don't want more, I want my son. No one seems to understand that. I want to tell him I'm sorry for the suffering I caused him. Until I can do that, I don't think the pain will ever go away.

# 2  Immediate Feelings

This chapter is about parents' feelings in the time immediately after their baby's death. Although each parent reacts individually, some reactions do seem to be shared by a great many parents. Many say that at first they were extremely shocked and found it hard to believe what had happened. Many also talk about a particular moment when they faced reality and took in the fact that their baby had died. All parents describe painful, overwhelming emotions, and above all, the pain and sadness of loss.

## 'IT CAN'T BE TRUE'

In the first minutes, hours or even days after their baby's death, parents often find themselves saying 'this can't be true', 'this can't be happening to us', 'it's a bad dream: soon we'll wake up'. They cannot believe what has happened. Tom and his partner, Rosalind, learnt that their baby had died during early labour:

> 'I had no idea how to react. I felt so detached from the whole business. I gazed out of the window and cuddled Rosalind as she wept. It was almost that I was imagining the whole affair . . .'

Rosalind had suffered an abrupted placenta and her labour was difficult and worrying. Tom was told that Rosalind's own life was in danger, and there was never any hope that the baby could be born alive. Even so, Tom found this hard to believe:

> 'As the end of the labour drew near, I nurtured a secret hope in my heart that they had all been wrong, that our baby would emerge alive and fighting for life. Should they be preparing an incubator in intensive care or something, I kept wondering — but did not dare ask.'

Many parents feel numbed by their baby's death. They feel unable to feel anything. They may cry, but still cannot accept that what is happening to them is real. And for some, disbelief is so strong that at first they do not cry. Carol, whose baby son was stillborn, writes:

> 'I was amazed at how calm and collected I was. My baby had died. I couldn't understand why I didn't break down, why I didn't throw myself about, weep and shout. I felt as though I was acting in a play. I was some other character and the real me was sitting in the audience and watching.'

Ian's baby died after six days in intensive care. Ian, too, had a feeling of detachment. He had to make all the arrangements for his son's funeral:

> 'Friends felt sorry for me because I had to do everything — see the funeral director, make all the phone calls, make the decisions. But I didn't find it so hard, because all the time I was doing these things, I wasn't thinking or feeling *anything*.'

In this state of shock and numbness, parents sometimes find themselves doing or thinking things that seem quite inappropriate, almost carrying on as normal, as though nothing terrible has happened:

> 'Even in the midst of it all, even while I was holding John in my arms and the tears were streaming down my face, I caught myself thinking, "What are we going to do with the cot and all the rest of the things we've bought?" I was upset to find myself thinking like that. But it was just as though there was a bit of my mind that hadn't taken hold of what was happening.'

The mind may *not* at first take hold of what is happening. For a while it seems to protect itself, refusing to take in something that is so hard to accept. 'I *knew* it was true but I couldn't *believe* it was true' is how one mother puts it. Mary L, who had felt particularly special during her pregnancy because she was expecting twins, describes the shock she felt when she discovered they had died in the womb and how, subconsciously, she continued to think that her babies were alive:

'The first night of knowing was the worst, I think, of my life. Everyone who has gone through it knows that the terrible trauma of losing the baby you are expecting is that all your emotions suddenly have to make an emergency stop and do a three-point turn. Pregnancy is all about life, hope, joyful anticipation of the future, happiness that other people share with you. To have it suddenly turned into its absolute opposite — death, sadness, darkness and despair — and to have to come to terms with that is the most unbearable torture. Every time I momentarily let go into shallow dream sleep, my mind reverted to the optimistic, special happiness I had felt. Then the part of it that knew the truth jerked me awake, to relive the awful truth, until it finally sunk in that I was now special in a very different sort of way.'

One reason why it can be so hard initially to believe that a baby has died is, as Mary says, because the death is often so unexpected and sudden. It is a complete reversal of all that parents have anticipated. To find birth and death brought this close together is confusing and shocking.

Jenny had a happy, straightforward pregnancy with no reason to expect anything to go wrong. When she went into labour three weeks early she was delighted. Her due date was just after Christmas and she had been hoping the birth would be earlier, so that she and the baby would be able to spend Christmas at home, along with her husband and 2½-year-old daughter:

'My labour started at 5 p.m. on the Sunday and I was extremely surprised at the speed and strength of the contractions which, from the onset, were occurring every minute. We left for the hospital, arriving at 6 p.m. I was firstly examined by a chirpy student midwife who attached belt monitors to me. However, she could not locate the fetal heart. "Don't worry," she said, "I am only a student. I'll get a senior midwife." I did not worry. After all, I was sure that I had just felt my baby kick twice. The senior midwife came and tried, however also without success. The doctor was called. Now I was worried. By the time he arrived, my contractions felt unbearable and these intensified once he had broken the waters. There was meconium present. I felt dazed. He attached an electrode monitor to the baby's head and also scanned me. Eventually, the doctor quietly told us that if the baby was still alive, he was very sick. This couldn't be happening to us. I felt like an actor on a surreal stage, taking part in an awful nightmare, saying lines, not believing, just feeling detached. Minutes later, the doctor said he could perform a caesarean but there really was no point.

'Our little boy was born at 7.02 p.m. I held him in my arms and stared at our perfectly-formed, albeit blue, baby and felt hopelessly empty. My husband held him and cried deeply. I was put in a side room in the antenatal ward and my husband stayed with me that night. I did not scream or cry hysterically, yet I could not sleep. I lay staring at the clock all night, hardly shedding a tear.'

In two short hours, all Jenny's hopes and expectations had been turned upside-down. She had gone into hospital delighted to be in labour and looking forward to the birth of her second child. Two hours later, the unimagined and unimaginable had happened — her baby son was dead:

'We were prepared for and expected great joy but within minutes were plummeted into desperate grief.'

Jenny's inability to believe what had happened continued in the week after her son's death:

'In a strange way, we clung to the feeling that he was still with us. We wanted and needed to see him again before finally saying goodbye.'

At the end of that week, she and her husband went back to the hospital to say goodbye to their baby. They had arranged a short, private service in the hospital chapel. It was then that they began to take in that their baby was truly dead:

'The horror of what had happened was beginning to seep in . . . To see that tiny coffin, no bigger than a shoe box, was dreadfully distressing.'

Like Jenny, Jacqui learnt during labour that her baby had died. She had not had an easy pregnancy and had suspected that things were not going well. When she was twenty-seven weeks pregnant, she was admitted to hospital with suspected premature labour. Although the labour was successfully suppressed with drugs, Jacqui still felt very unwell and was convinced something was wrong. Then, when she was thirty-three weeks pregnant, she became ill. She was violently sick and had strong abdominal pains. Her GP examined her and tried unsuccessfully to find her baby's heartbeat. He sent her to hospital:

'By the time I arrived at hospital, I felt considerably worse. I was sick again and I began to bleed profusely. I was very frightened and sensed that something was terribly wrong. They tried desperately to find a heartbeat on the scanner. In the end, I had to ask for confirmation of what I already knew. The registrar held my hand and gently explained that the baby had died — probably many hours before.'

Jacqui's labour was induced, and after twelve difficult hours, her son was born:

'He was very beautiful, and I felt very elated to have given birth.'

Jacqui knew that her baby had died before her labour was induced. In fact, she knew even before she was told by the registrar. And she had suspected that something was wrong much earlier in her pregnancy. But believing that her baby had died was still very hard. She describes how, after her son's birth, she and her husband had spent time with their baby:

'We didn't think of him as being not alive, but sleeping peacefully. We enjoyed getting to know our baby. Then, after a brief drugged sleep, I awoke to find my husband asleep in a chair beside me. I remember thinking, "Where is our baby? Why isn't he here with us?" It was not until I heard other babies crying that the awful truth dawned on me — my baby did not cry because he was dead.'

The shock of a baby's death is often made much worse because the events surrounding the death happen with such drama and speed. The death happens as a crisis. Jacqui, for example, like many other mothers, heard the news of her baby's death when she was in pain, distressed, and in the midst of an emergency. However, for other parents it happens differently. Some know days or even weeks in advance that their baby will die or will be born dead. And sometimes a baby's death — on a neonatal unit, for example — happens very peacefully. Alison and Neil's baby daughter, Rose, died in intensive care when she was three weeks old. They had been told the day after she was born that she would not live:

'When she died, we accepted it. But when we were first told that there was no hope for her, that was something we really couldn't accept.

We thought they must have got it wrong. Especially because for some while after they gave us the news, she began to look better. She even put on a bit of weight. The week after they told us was the worst time. We were hoping against hope. We were willing her to live, even though we knew it was hopeless. We'd lost our baby, yet she hadn't died.'

Catherine too found it hard to believe that her baby son would die. He was diagnosed as having hypoplastic left heart syndrome just a few days after he was born, and she was told that he would not live long:

'I knew that if I was going to make anything of whatever time I had with Ben then I had to accept that he was going to die. But I also felt that if I *did* accept it, if I let myself believe what they were telling me, then I would somehow make it happen. If I refused to believe it, then maybe it wouldn't happen.'

Even parents who, like Catherine, watch their baby's condition slowly worsen day by day, may still find it hard to accept their baby's death when it happens. A period of hours, days or even weeks is simply not enough time for anybody to prepare themselves for such a complete reversal of all that they wanted, hoped for and looked forward to:

'I'd never seen anyone die, I'd never seen a dead body, I'd never been bereaved. How could I be prepared? Anyway, I didn't *want* to be prepared. I didn't want my baby to die.'

## FACING REALITY

'We had to face reality: our baby had died, and so had all the great plans we had made.'

For many parents there comes a particular moment when their baby's death becomes real to them. They take in fully what has happened for the first time and admit to themselves that there is no escaping the hurt and the grief. This realisation is not necessarily immediate — though for Rosalind, it came as soon as her daughter was born. From the moment she was told that her baby had died inside her, she felt devastated. But the devastation was unfocused, 'as if the pregnancy had been cancelled and I didn't understand why':

'I knew there would be a dead baby when I gave birth, but somehow it didn't register that it was really my little baby that had died. I cried throughout labour of course, but the real, tearing agony only began when she was born. I'd had three babies before and I knew how people should react in that marvellous instant when you push them out to face the world. She was born to silence, and the doctors and midwives all cried, bless their hearts, and someone told me it was a girl. It really hit me then — my daughter, my longed-for baby daughter was dead, and nothing would ever be the same. It wasn't just an aborted pregnancy, it was my dear little girl. I wouldn't wish that moment on anybody, it's so terribly hard to come to terms with birth and death together. I wanted to feed her, to see what colour her eyes were, to show her to my other children, and all I could do was hold her and count the minutes till they took her from me.'

For some parents, the reality of their baby's death does not become absolutely clear to them for a long time — perhaps not until they hold a funeral and their baby is cremated or buried, or perhaps even later. For Sandra, whose baby Terri Jean was stillborn, realisation came when she left the hospital without her baby.

When she and her husband arrived at the hospital, Sandra was examined and was told that she was 4 cm dilated:

'Then the moment of truth came. There was no heartbeat. Four different doctors examined me and all failed to find a heartbeat. The pains were stronger than ever and I was asked if I wanted something to ease them, but I didn't want anything. We still hadn't been told the baby was dead. I was crying and I said, "The baby is dead, isn't it?" and was answered with a very quiet "Yes, it looks that way." My husband and I were heartbroken and just cried and cried.

'I remember telling my husband to get my mum. All I knew was that I wanted her there with me. While he was gone, I thought I was dreaming, having a nightmare, and that I would wake up and everything would be all right. It wasn't.

'At 2 a.m. I was still lying on the bed and by now my husband, mum and dad were all with me. At 6.30 a.m. my waters broke and I asked how long it would be before the baby was born. They said it wouldn't be much longer. All the time, in the back of my mind, my baby was not dead: it couldn't be, because we wanted the baby so much. I was full term, the pregnancy had gone well, so what could have happened?

'At 7.44 a.m. I gave birth to a beautiful, dark-haired baby girl. The midwife asked me if I wanted to hold her. Of course I did, she was my baby, I had waited nine months for her. I held her gently in my arms and the nurse took a photograph of her. We named her Terri Jean. The nurse dressed her in a white nightgown and a nappy and put her in a cot with a blanket as if she were alive.

'At 11.30 a.m. the nurse came and asked if she could take the baby away now and we agreed. I asked if I could go straight home. We packed my things back in the case and left. As we left the room, I walked past another room and the door was open and I could see my baby in her cot, the room was dark and I felt heartbroken. I just couldn't stand any more of this nightmare. As we came out into the car-park, I broke down. I had come to the hospital with a baby and now I was going home without one.

'When I got home, I just sat in the chair crying for hours and hours and I couldn't speak. I remember going upstairs and seeing all the baby clothes and other things. The clothes were so tiny and I held them to me and cried all over again. It seemed like it was years ago, but it was only a few hours.'

For Sandra, events were very rapid. The experience can be very different for parents whose babies live for days or weeks. They may know for a long time in advance that their baby is likely to die. So for them, truth dawns in a more gradual, though no less painful, way. Gillian and Carl's baby, Christopher, lived for eleven days. He was born prematurely at twenty-eight weeks, and rushed immediately to the nearest neonatal unit — in a hospital 100 miles away. After twenty-four hours, Gillian and Carl were able to follow him:

'We juggled fears and facts. He was a good weight . . . but he was breathing badly. He was twenty-eight weeks . . . but he had to endure that long journey to the new hospital. He was loved and wanted so very much . . . but so very weak. We prayed.'

Over the days that followed, Gillian and Carl went from hope to despair to hope again, until finally it became clear that there was no hope left. At first, Christopher seemed to be doing well:

'Although he was sick, everyone was optimistic. Progress was going to be slow, but he was responding to treatment. All we had to do was be patient. After a previous miscarriage, years of trying, five threatened miscarriages in this pregnancy and months of anxious waiting, we had a son. We were over the moon.

'Then, disaster. He blew a hole in his already fragile lungs. He had to be operated on immediately and a drain inserted into his lung. The operation was to take place in the room where he was. We asked to stay. There were doubts. They didn't want us fainting or panicking. We assured them we wouldn't. We "scrubbed up". I held Chris's hand, and Carl, my husband and his dad, held mine. We all survived.'

The following day a hole developed in Christopher's other lung and the same operation had to be repeated. The next day, there was yet another hole, and this time Christopher's heart stopped as well. He survived — but Gillian and Carl were now told that their baby was dying. They were advised that if there was no improvement soon, it would be time to think of switching off the machines:

'No words can describe how utterly wretched and empty we felt. It was beyond belief. We wanted to cry and shout and sob and deny it but we knew we had to hang on. "Chin up for Chrissy" was our motto. We decided to give him a good talking to. One on each side of the incubator, each holding a hand, we told him precisely what we thought. We willed him to live and it worked. His next blood test was miraculously better. The machines stayed on!

'He continued to improve. Again there was optimism. A good day followed. I was even allowed to wipe his bottom and put a clean nappy under him. I felt like a real mother! Our spirits lifted. We actually thought about the future and the time we would take him home.'

But the next day there was another crisis, another hole, another operation, another drain. Gillian and Carl felt they were still 'in with a chance', but now only a slim one. And when Christopher was ten days old, that chance disappeared. The consultant told them that Christopher was dying. If the ventilator was switched off, he would be dead within seconds. If it was left on, his heart would eventually fail — probably within hours. They decided to keep the ventilator on and to wait:

'Later that night the consultant told us that Chris now needed a cuddle and a love. She said that she would arrange to keep him "wired up" while we held him. He was under sedation, paralysed by drugs, in no pain, and we could see that he was indeed fading. We cuddled him until he died — nine hours later. Just before he died, he managed to open his eyes and one tear tumbled down his cheek. It was as though he was saying goodbye.'

For Gillian and Carl, there was no questioning the reality of Christopher's death: they were very much part of it. Afterwards, though feeling very sad and deprived, they also described themselves as 'lucky' because 'we had him for eleven precious days. Even from so short a time we have a store of memories.'

Other parents, often those whose babies never lived outside the womb, are left with very few memories and can find it much more difficult to take in the reality of their loss. Those who never saw their baby or who had very little contact with him or her perhaps find it hardest of all. When Peter and Sallie's son, James, was delivered just a few days short of twenty-eight weeks gestation, Peter was asked to leave the delivery room. So he did not see his son until he was in an incubator in the neonatal unit. Then, because he had a cold, Peter could not risk touching James. He was afraid that he would pass on the infection.

Ten days later, James died. Peter and Sallie were called to the hospital in the early morning and when they arrived, James's tubes had already been removed. Sallie held her son for the first time since his birth, and she and Peter were given a room where they could spend time with him. Sallie writes:

'Peter did not want to hold him at first but eventually he did, and then he cried and said, "This makes him real." All week he had not touched his little son.'

## 'IT'S ALL SO CRUEL'

Many different feelings come to parents in the time immediately after their baby's death — anger, outrage, fear, guilt, bitterness, utter despair. Above all, there is overwhelming sadness. This sadness is hard to bear because it carries with it the certain knowledge that there is nothing that can be done about it. Nothing can bring back the pregnancy that has ended or the baby who has died. Trying to accept this hard fact, trying to accept the unacceptable, is a long and weary job. At the beginning, it is agonising.

Feelings can be violent, intense, extreme — sometimes frighteningly so. Some parents, particularly if this is the first major crisis in their lives or the first time that someone close to them has died, are shocked to discover the strength of their reactions. Jean, for example, who was in her early twenties when her first baby died, says that until that time she had had a very easy, happy life. When her baby died, just eight days after the birth, she was devastated not only because she had lost the baby she had loved and wanted, but also because her whole understanding of life was turned upside down:

> 'I felt as though I'd fallen into a gaping black hole. It seemed as though the world was suddenly a different place where terrible things could happen without reason or warning. I didn't want to live in a world like that.'

Like Jean, many parents describe desolation and despair. They feel 'set apart', singled out, punished and very lonely. The longing for their baby can be overwhelming, and the feeling of deprivation is like the after-effects of a stunning physical blow. Some parents feel frightened — by their experience of death, by the strength of their own feelings and of facing the world again. They may feel they have no future:

> 'The emptiness of it all was terrible. I wanted to die. Life seemed utterly pointless.'

Many parents feel anger and hatred towards themselves, towards the doctors and nurses, towards God or fate:

> 'It would have helped me, just at that particular time, if I could have done something violent to express how violent I felt. I was cooped up in my hospital room, feeling physically very weak, consumed with anger and hate. I hated my body because it had failed me. I hated my breasts for producing milk when there was no baby to feed. I hated the doctor who had failed to revive my baby after she was born. I hated all those women who had live, healthy babies to feed and care for. I hated the sad faces of people who came to see me. Most of all, I hated God for letting this awful, unimaginable thing happen . . .'

Tim too felt angry after a scan showed that his baby had died. He describes being in the hospital after receiving the news of his baby's death:

> 'It was incredibly awful to be in that place, surrounded by mothers about to give birth, other fathers waiting, and the medical staff just carrying on as normal. I had this overwhelming feeling I wanted to shock someone — to shout at the mothers sitting there nine months pregnant, lighting up a last cigarette and thinking to themselves, "How sweet, his wife's in there having a baby." I wanted to shout at them, "My baby's dead." I wanted to shock them all, but you can't.'

Sometimes parents feel some kind of anger towards each other. When something terrible has happened, it is natural enough to look for someone to blame. Often we pin blame on the very person we love or need the most:

> 'It was as though I wanted to make sure that Geoff was as hurt as I was. I said something that I shall never be able to forgive myself for. I said, "You never wanted this baby anyway." It wasn't true.'

There is a lot of bewilderment in this kind of anger. It is bewildering that birth and death should be brought so close together. It seems senseless, beyond understanding, a complete reversal of all that has been expected and hoped for. 'Such a waste,' one mother said about her baby son's death, 'such a bloody waste.'

Many parents feel that they are to blame for their baby's death. Some think back to something particular they did and feel sure that if only they hadn't done it their baby would still be alive. Some feel to blame in a more general way. They feel that their baby was a part of themselves. Without them, he or she would not have lived; so without them, he or she would surely not have died. Feeling responsible for their baby's death can mean that parents also take the blame for their own or each other's heartache, and maybe also for the heartache which the death has caused to others — to their own parents, for example, or their other children.

For women especially, feelings of responsibility can be very strong. They, after all, have carried and cared for their baby throughout pregnancy. When their baby dies, they may feel they have not 'cared' enough:

'I feel guilty because Amy relied on me to be able to survive and because she depended on me I feel responsible for her death.'

Other women blame themselves because they had not wanted to be pregnant in the first place, or perhaps had not felt entirely positive about their pregnancy in some other way. When their baby dies, it may seem as though the tragedy is somehow the result of their negative feelings. They may feel that they are being 'punished'. They may feel remorse because only after their baby's death do they realise just how much they loved and wanted him or her.

Many women feel that they have failed. They feel that they should have been able to have a healthy, 'successful' pregnancy, a normal, 'successful' labour, and a live, healthy baby, because so many hundreds and thousands of other women 'succeed' in doing these things. Connie says:

'The one thing that society would have you believe all women can do, you can't.'

Some women speak of failing themselves, some of failing others. Bridgette said that when her husband held their dead baby:

'I felt so sorry for him. I felt I had failed him badly.'

For parents whose baby dies after some days or weeks, there can be recriminations and feelings of guilt as they look back over their baby's short life. Some feel they did not spend enough time by the incubator or cot, that they didn't talk enough, touch and stroke enough, or do enough for their baby. Others have particular regrets about something they did not say or do — a cuddly toy that was never given, a story that was never read — and their feelings of sadness become concentrated on this omission. Sometimes there are feelings that the baby would have lived if only they, the parents, had just hoped for it, prayed for it or willed it more strongly.

All these first feelings are very cruel. To bereaved parents, it seems at first that they will be destroyed by their grief. It seems impossible to feel so much and to survive. Very gradually, over time, feelings change, and although nothing may be forgotten, the pain slowly softens and becomes more bearable. It is grieving which helps to bring this about.

## THE NEED TO GRIEVE

'People tried to comfort me. My family and friends were wonderful really and did all they could to help me. But what they couldn't understand was that even though I felt so desperate, I didn't want to be comforted or made to feel better. I didn't want even one tiny bit of the pain to be taken away because . . . it was the only thing I had left.'

This is what grieving is like at first. It is almost a matter of making the pain worse in order to make it better. Sarah, whose baby died after a week in intensive care, says:

'For a long time, I put off crying. I found I could actually hold back the tears. I knew the thoughts that would make me cry, and I could stop myself from thinking them. I was frightened of hurting myself any more. But then I found that if I let myself cry, it was awful but so awful that afterwards I felt a bit better for a while.'

Like Sarah, Sallie was initially so shocked that she seemed to have no feelings. Then, after a while, she found that it helped her if she allowed herself to think about her baby and dwell on her memories. This is how she describes the time immediately after her son's death, from the moment of leaving the neonatal unit where he died:

'Eventually, about 11 a.m., we had to leave the hospital. We left James in the sister's arms and she promised me she would look after him. We gave permission for a post-mortem.

'When we got home, my mother was sitting in the garden. She knew James had died because Peter had phoned her from the hospital, but I hadn't spoken to her. I went to her in the garden and I said, "I'm sorry Mum." I was dry-eyed.

'I can't remember anything about the rest of that day. It's a fog. But I know I didn't cry. Later, in the evening, I was sitting upstairs on the edge of the bed and suddenly I started to scream. I screamed and screamed. Both Peter and my mother were very alarmed and didn't know what to do . . .

'We had James's funeral six days after that and Peter went back to work a few days after the funeral. I was at home on my own then. I had a lot of friends who came to see me and be with me, but I was on my own a lot too. I would listen to music. There was a particular piece that helped me to think about James and I played it over and over again. I looked at the photo we had of James. I wrote letters to people, telling them about what had happened or replying to their letters. And I wrote down an account of everything that happened in James's short life. I wanted to do that straight away so I would never forget and he would never be forgotten. I sent a copy of what I'd written to everyone in the family.'

But for some parents it is very difficult to begin to grieve. Many, often encouraged by family, friends and others, do their best to 'put their experience behind them', to forget and get on with life. Jan, for example, was desolate after her son's death, but she had no chance to express how she felt. She had miscarried when she was six months pregnant:

'The whole experience was tidied away as rapidly as possible. In hospital, the staff behaved as though it had simply never happened. And because it had been so traumatic, I felt relieved to tidy it away too. I came out of hospital the next day and I carried on as normal. My friends didn't want to talk about it: they found it too difficult. Robin and I talked with each other, but not to anybody else.

'I was determined to get pregnant again. When my daughter was born a year later, I felt as though I had come back to life. I was fine. A year after that, I became terribly ill. They could find nothing wrong with me, but I was sick every day, I couldn't eat, I couldn't even sit up — I had to lie down most of the time. I thought that I was dying.

'I think that it can take a long time to express emotions, but in the end they have to be expressed, even if your body has to take over and do it for you.'

Grieving is the way we express feelings of loss. By expressing these feelings, we come to understand them better and deal with them. Then, gradually, the pain lessens. So in their own way and in their own time, parents need to be able to let out their feelings. To be able to grieve, there has to be something to grieve over. Parents need memories and mementos. They also need opportunities to grieve. When they are denied these things, as Jan was, grieving becomes very difficult, and sometimes it is left undone.

In Chapter 4 we look at grief and grieving in much more detail. In the next chapter, we look at parents' experiences in hospital because it is clear that the way parents are treated at the time of their baby's death can have far-reaching consequences, for good or ill.

# 3 Experiences in Hospital

This chapter describes parents' experiences in hospital and looks at what professionals can do to care for and support parents when their baby dies. Some parents receive sensitive, high-quality care in hospital, but others are less fortunate, and some parents, who receive very poor hospital care, feel distressed and angry for a long time afterwards. What is written in this chapter cannot change what these parents have experienced, but we draw on their experiences to describe parents' needs at the time of their baby's death, and to suggest how hospital care can, where necessary, be improved.

## 'I'LL NEVER FORGET'

Most parents have very vivid memories of their baby's death and all the events surrounding it. Years, even a lifetime later many can still clearly remember the details of what happened, what was said and done, and what they thought and felt. Particular sights or sounds or smells can bring the memories flooding back.

In the weeks and months immediately after their baby's death, parents often use their memories to re-live their experience over and over again. Doing this is sad and painful, but it can also be helpful and is a part of grieving. Some parents write down everything that happened; some talk about it; some simply re-live their experiences in their thoughts. One mother describes the process as 'like watching your own private, personal video'.

For most parents, remembering their baby's death means remembering what happened in hospital. So inevitably, the way they feel about the hospital and the hospital staff colours their memories. If they feel that they were well cared for, they have at least some positive memories among their unhappy ones. But parents who feel they were badly cared for can be left with an unnecessary, extra layer of distress. They are likely to feel that distress every time they think about their baby, and often it clouds their memories and complicates their grieving.

Joanne and Jeremy, and their baby, Jason, received very good hospital care. Jason was taken to the special care baby unit immediately he was born. He lived for eleven days. His story illustrates what an enormous difference good hospital care can make:

'Throughout our time on SCBU [the special care baby unit] the staff were magnificent in their support. They gave us comfort through our tears, spent time talking our worst fears through, and created a "family" environment in which Jeremy was made to feel a vital part as the father of Jason. Without their support we would have been so lonely and lost in our distress, so abandoned. They gave me time alone but I always knew that they were there, and Jeremy was assured that he could ring any time during the night to check on Jason if he wanted to or even sleep on the unit to be near his son.

'I really don't think there can be anything more horrifying than to have your own baby breathe his last breath in your arms. Fortunately, the sister in charge that night rang us in time for us to get to him before he died. It had been my first day home.

'We were surrounded by the nurses who had cared for him and the doctor, all giving their support and sympathy which helped us enormously, and also made us feel that our little mite was important to them too, that he had been genuinely loved by others as well as by us. It meant a great deal to us that the nurses were able to shed tears with us, that as the care-givers they didn't need a stiff upper lip or some kind of professional stoicism. It helped us both to let our own feelings go in that most harrowing of moments. One of the nurses baptised Jason as I held him. We weren't regular church members but it was vital to us that he had this baptism — I am so glad that the nurses remembered as it was the last thing on my mind at that time.

'After Jason had died, the sister in charge gently suggested we might like to take Jason into one of the rooms where we could be alone with him. I was hesitant about this, I wasn't sure if it was the right thing to do, whilst deep in my heart I just didn't want to let him go. Fortunately, they had the experience to know that this would be a good idea for us, and we were encouraged to spend some time alone with him. This time we spent with our baby was one of the most important and precious of times for us. At last that awful feeding tube was removed, at last the oxygen mask wasn't needed, at last I could cuddle, kiss and hold my baby with no tubes or monitors, no worries of anything further happening to him. He was released from his misery and I could carry him out of the hot nursery, my baby and me together at last.

'Jeremy and I grieved so deeply for our little boy, we took photos and felt we didn't want to let him go, but the cooler he became the more we were able to accept that he had truly left us. The staff checked on us about every twenty minutes, respecting our privacy but also showing us they were still there supporting us. Eventually, they came to bathe him and change his clothes and asked me if I would like to do it. I decided that I wanted to do everything that I could for him. I had never bathed him — I wanted this one chance, he was my baby, I would care for him until the end. After I'd bathed him the nurses offered us a lovely white robe to dress him in. He looked so serene and peaceful, as if asleep, in his cot.

'Before we left the SCBU that terrible night, the staff assured us that if at any time we wanted to see Jason, day or night, we could come down and they would bring him to us. That was very reassuring. It meant we didn't have to feel we'd said goodbye to him for the last time. They also said that if we needed to talk to anyone, day or night, that they were always there for us, ready to listen, to help, either by phone or if we wanted to visit. Our important connection with the SCBU did not end after Jason had died — their support continued and we were especially touched when so many nurses came to Jason's funeral. We have since been back to visit Jason's "home" many times.'

Sensitive, supportive care such as Joanne and Jeremy received cannot take away pain; it cannot even soften grief. But it changes the way loss is felt, and it can make grieving easier. It means that among all the painful feelings and memories, there are also some good things to remember — people's kindness, concern and understanding, most especially — and the feeling that something of great importance was done properly and well.

In recent years, hospital care for parents whose baby dies has improved dramatically. There is much greater understanding of what it means to lose a baby, so there is also much greater understanding of what parents need in the way of care and support. But even now, this does not mean that good care and support are always provided. Angela H was acutely distressed by the way she was treated in hospital. Her daughter, Victoria, was born prematurely and lived for just over twelve hours:

'They wouldn't let me go down to the special unit to see her because I was strapped up with drips. After nattering them, they finally brought her to see me and I held her for ten minutes. One of the midwives was with me and she made me feel guilty each time I touched her. But Victoria knew I was there and moved her fingers when I touched them. I asked a nurse later if Victoria knew who I was but she said no. This made me upset.

'When they had brought her for me to see me, they only gave her one hour to live, but she proved to them and me she was a fighter because she lived four and a half hours longer.

'The sister of the special unit was very snappy with me, especially when she asked me whether I wanted her christened or not, which I did. Also, when I asked the nurses how she was doing, most of them said she shouldn't live much longer, as though I was waiting for her to die. When she did die, the sister of the special unit just stuck her head round the door and said, "Your baby died fifteen minutes ago and I've washed and dressed her." Then she shut the door. Five minutes later a nurse came in and I was in a right state. I was shaking and really upset, and she said, "Never mind, you can have some more, and maybe it's for the best anyway."

'The sister of the ward was going to arrange for me and Barry and my mother to go and see Victoria and spend as long as we wanted with her, alone. But again there was someone there all the time, and she told us to go as there was nothing else to do. This again upset me as Victoria was mine and Barry's daughter, but the way they carried on she was just another baby.'

To be left with memories like these and, just as upsetting, to be left *without* the memories that are needed, makes loss and grieving very hard. Since parents do not forget, they need to feel as good as they possibly can about what they remember. If their memories cause them to feel upset or angry, then remembering becomes much more painful. Long-term bitterness can be added to a lifelong grief.

## WHAT DO PARENTS NEED?

Parents' experiences in hospital make it clear what kind of hospital care can help them. First, they need to be treated respectfully by those who care for and come into contact with them. They also need to be able to take part in what happens to them and to their baby, making their own decisions whenever possible and if they wish to do so. They need to be given information. And lastly, they need to be given time.

## RESPECT

It makes a very great difference to parents if they are treated with respect by the professionals who care for them. They need respect for themselves, for their baby, and for all that they are going through. In other words, they need to feel that they matter.

Sue R and her husband, Peter, were given this kind of respect. Their daughter, Naomi, was born when Sue was twenty-five weeks pregnant and lived for just twenty minutes:

> 'The hospital staff made us feel that this was not just a non-event to be forgotten about. Even though we had not got a live baby, Naomi was important. The sister stressed that we had two daughters, Lois, then aged 3, and Naomi; and encouraged us to think positively about Naomi, as someone we would never forget.
>
> 'Immediately prior to her birth, the sister told us the baby would not live and we appreciated her honesty. They dressed her in a gown and let me hold her for as long as I wanted; she in fact died in my arms. Sister offered to take a photo of her, and we gratefully accepted. We were allowed to stay in the delivery room for as long as we wanted, and it was up to us when we wanted to say "goodbye" to Naomi and hand her over to the staff. Peter, Naomi and I were left on our own for at least an hour and the staff just popped their head round the door occasionally to see if we needed anything. They really got the balance between helpfulness and privacy exactly right. During that time we were offered the use of the hospital phone to call our family.
>
> 'We were told the rest of the staff on duty wanted to see Naomi, and this added to our feeling that she was important and not a failure because she'd not survived. We were made to feel proud of her and she was always referred to by name. One of the midwives who helped to deliver her came back about an hour later very red-eyed. It helped us to know that the staff themselves were moved by our circumstances. The sister offered more than once to call the hospital chaplain for us, but as it was past 10.30 p.m. we didn't want to disturb his sleep. But the offer was appreciated. After we had parted with Naomi we were told we could see her at any time, and the sister described how she would appear to put our minds at rest.'

Sadly, some parents' experiences are very different. When Pauline's baby died, no one showed that they cared:

> 'When I was seven months pregnant, they discovered that my baby was dead and I was induced. Because the baby was dead, they gave me a lot of pain-killers, but it was a long labour. I delivered a baby

boy. I don't remember much else about the delivery but just the midwife telling me that I had had a boy. They took him away and I didn't see him.

'I was allowed home two days later. I was on my own a lot during that time and felt very lonely and sad. The doctor only came to see me once and told me nothing about my baby. I felt that I couldn't ask. I don't know how my baby has been disposed of or what they would have done to him. I feel so lost and out of touch, as though I don't really matter and haven't got a say in anything any more.'

It can be very hurtful for anyone to find that a major crisis in their lives is treated by others as a minor event. It can be confusing too, because it seems to suggest that it isn't a major crisis after all. Pauline, like all parents, needed the hospital staff to recognise the importance of her baby's death, yet it was treated as little more than a medical incident.

Showing respect means recognising and acknowledging the importance of a baby's death — and of parents' loss. It also means caring for parents as individuals, and responding sensitively to their individual feelings and needs. All too often, assumptions are made about what parents want. Instead, parents need the chance to express their wishes, knowing that the professionals caring for them will not judge them for what they say and will try hard to meet their needs.

Often, of course, it is difficult for parents to know what they want: they are shocked and distressed, probably bewildered by the speed of events, and many have never dealt with death before. So sometimes, parents need staff to talk things over with them, to make suggestions and help them work out what is right for them. Sometimes, too, they need space in which to change their minds. They may need to reconsider decisions made in the first few hours or even days after their baby's death, because it takes time to feel clear about what they want and need. A lot of parents are left with regrets because they were not given a second chance to say what they did or didn't want.

Respect is due not only to parents but also to their baby. Parents appreciate it enormously if staff handle their baby as tenderly as if he or she was alive, call him or her by name and show, in every possible way, that their baby is important and immensely valuable. It is essential that parents are informed and consulted about everything that is decided for or done to their baby, and whenever possible their wishes should be followed. The feelings that come with parenthood do not die when the baby dies, and parents need ways of expressing their feelings. Taking part in decisions and arrangements, and maybe caring for their baby's body after death (for example, washing and dressing their baby), are all important.

Sometimes parents are caused distress because staff behave as though the baby belongs to them, or to the hospital. Many parents write about being 'allowed' to hold their dead baby for a certain time, and staff then taking the baby away. After this, parents may not see their baby again. Yet there is no reason why parents should not have the amount of time that they themselves feel they want and need with their baby. And later on, there is no reason why the body cannot be brought back from the mortuary, if that is what parents wish, so that they can see their baby again. Many parents, who would like to see their baby a second or third time, feel unable to ask, but they should not have to do so: staff should offer this possibility.

Finally, one very simple way in which professionals — and everyone concerned — can show respect is to show that they care: the words 'I'm sorry' can express sadness and sympathy, and mean a great deal. Those who do show they care give something to parents which is out of all proportion to the effort involved.

## TAKING PART, MAKING DECISIONS

Hospital staff can all too easily take over when a baby dies. Often they do so with the intention of sparing parents pain. But by taking over, they can take away from parents their experience of their baby's death. Even though it is painful, parents need to be able to take part in what happens to them. They need to 'live it' as fully as possible, in their own way and at their own pace. This gives them a reality to believe in (not just a bad dream), and also memories which will help them to hold on to that reality over the months and years to come. Afterwards, they can look back on something that they experienced and that was really 'theirs', instead of on something that merely happened to them.

At a time when so much is beyond their control, parents also need to feel that they have at least some say in what is happening. Although they cannot prevent their baby's death, they can make choices about much that happens around the death, and afterwards. It is important that hospital staff and hospital systems allow parents the opportunity to be involved.

Lesley's baby died in her womb when she was thirty-five weeks pregnant. Lesley had been worried for several days because her baby seemed to be kicking less often. She went to her GP, who assured her that all was well. Two days later, at a hospital check-up, no heartbeat could be found:

'The doctor said I could be admitted immediately, but I didn't want that. He found a quiet room where we could talk; he held my hand and a nurse came with some tea. He asked me what I felt I wanted and I said I needed some time — I was so shocked and sad. They suggested I should go home and come back after the weekend, and that's what I chose to do.

'For me, that weekend was important: I had two last precious days with Louise still safe and loved inside me. In between our tears, Paul and I talked a lot and prepared ourselves to say goodbye. When Monday came, we went back to the hospital with our camera and some carefully chosen baby clothes. We explained how, if possible, we wanted the birth to be. I was induced that morning and Louise was born just after 3 p.m. We spent the rest of the day with her, cuddling her for the first and last time.'

Lesley was greatly helped by the feeling that she had some control over what was happening to her and to her baby. She was taking part and was not taken over, either by events or by other people.

Professionals sometimes seem to feel that they should protect parents from the stress of making decisions, and it is true that making decisions at a time of crisis and while in acute distress is far from easy. In addition, some of the decisions which bereaved parents face are very large and difficult decisions, which they never expected to have to make and which they are therefore quite unprepared for. But these are also decisions which are crucially important for parents and which they will live with for the rest of their lives. They do not need to be 'let off' making them. Instead, they need to be given time to think, talk and make up their minds, and they need sensitive help and support.

For Jill, the first hint that anything could be wrong came when she was examined in the labour ward and her doctors had difficulty in finding a heartbeat. Five hours later, her baby, Jessica, was stillborn:

'After she was born, she was offered to me to hold, but I refused. All I wanted them to do was take her away. I didn't want anything to do with her. I just wanted to wallow in my own grief.

'Eventually, as the second day after the birth came round, one particular nurse who was absolutely great with me, produced two photographs and asked me if I wanted to see my little girl. At first my answer was definitely no, but after she left I started thinking, who did she look like? what colour hair did she have? I had to know. After all, she was mine.

'I called the nurse back and asked to see the photos. I looked: it was the hardest thing I have ever done in my life. I saw my little girl fast asleep in a pretty little dress with flowers all around her head, in a lovely moses basket. I hadn't imagined how beautiful she would be.

'Then the next step came: did we want to go and see her? Yes, I said, but my husband was not too sure. But just as we were setting off, he stood up. "I want to come," he said. So we went, and there she was, absolutely beautiful. My little girl. Perfect.

'Eventually I had to leave her, very, very sad but glad for the chance to see exactly what she looked like.'

Like many other parents, it took Jill and her husband some time to know what they wanted and needed to do. Fortunately, they were given that time, and also the help they needed to reach a decision. The decision-making was not taken out of their hands.

## Decisions in which parents should be involved after the death of their baby

- When the baby is known to have died in the womb, parents should be able to take part in decisions about how labour and delivery will be managed. This includes decisions about whether and when the mother should be induced. Some women will choose to be induced as soon as possible, but others want time in which to collect their thoughts and prepare themselves as best they can for the loss of their baby. Some women wish, if possible, to avoid induction and wait for their labour to begin naturally. Mothers should also be involved in decisions about pain relief, position for delivery, whether they wish to hold their baby straight away or later, and all other aspects of their care during labour and delivery.

● When a baby has been born alive but it is known that he or she will certainly die, parents may wish to take their baby home (either for a short time or to die at home, depending on what parents want and what support is available).

● When a baby is known to be dying, parents should be involved in deciding whether and when life support is withdrawn. To do this, they need to be informed and supported by medical and nursing staff.

● It is important for parents to be able to choose whether, when and how often they want to see, hold and be with their dead baby.

● Parents should be able to choose what photographs are taken of their baby (for example, how the baby is dressed, whether the baby is held by the parents and/or in a moses basket, and so on).

● Unless there are overriding medical reasons, the mother herself should be able to decide the length of her hospital stay.

● Parents' permission for a post-mortem examination should always be asked for (regardless of the gestational age of their baby).

● Parents should be able to decide what kind of funeral or other ceremony they wish to have for their baby, and whether they wish to have their baby's body buried or cremated.

Some of these decisions are among the most difficult that people ever have to make. Many parents need support in making them — and in carrying them through. They need time to think, because they may only gradually become clear about their own wishes and needs. And they need information in order that their decisions can be informed not just by their own feelings but also by facts.

## INFORMATION

It is impossible to overemphasize the importance of information to parents. At a time of crisis, information gives strength and understanding, whereas to be deprived of information is disempowering and adds to parents' distress. They need information about what may happen, is happening, or has happened, to them and to their baby. They need to know about what choices they have, and how to make those choices. And they need information about practical matters, procedures and arrangements.

Parents cannot begin to understand what is happening or has happened to them or to their baby unless they are given the information they need. And if they cannot come to any understanding of what has happened, they cannot even begin to accept it. It is vital that hospital staff share fully with parents all that is known about their baby's death and, just as important, share honestly what is not known or understood.

Michelle lost her baby when she was thirty-one weeks pregnant. Her experience was made worse because she was not given the information or discussion she needed:

'On reaching the hospital, I was put straight onto a monitor. The doctor gave me an internal examination and saw that I was not dilating and decided to put me on a drip. I was very frightened and I got no explanation of what was happening. The baby's heartbeat was regular but the contractions were getting weaker. By 6.15 p.m. I was told by another doctor that I had to go into theatre for a caesarean section, totally unaware of what was happening. My baby was born at 6.42 p.m. and was rushed to the special care baby unit and died one and a half hours later.

'I later learned, when I was leaving hospital, that the placenta had come away from my womb prematurely. I never got any explanation of why such things happen or what could have caused it. They performed a post-mortem on the baby and found nothing. On leaving hospital, I searched through the libraries trying to find an answer that would satisfy me. All I found was information on miscarriages in the first four months of pregnancy, and most books just brushed on abruption of the placenta. Because I cannot find any information that would put my mind at ease, I believe I may have been to blame for my baby's death . . .'

A certain amount of information can and should be given to parents at the time of or just after their baby's death and before they leave the hospital. But all parents should also be given a follow-up appointment at the hospital some weeks later. When a post-mortem has been carried out, the follow-up appointment is usually arranged to take place when the post-mortem results are available, normally about four to six weeks after the death. Although it can be hard for parents to wait this long for information and discussion which is so badly needed, the delay can give them time to sort out and perhaps write down the questions they want to ask.

At the appointment, parents should be given as much information as possible about the events leading up to their baby's death, and about the death itself. The results of the post-mortem (if one has been performed) should be carefully explained. And parents should have the opportunity to ask questions and discuss their concerns with the professionals who were involved in their own and their baby's care. (Information about the implications of their baby's death for a future pregnancy is also extremely important for most parents. This is discussed in Chapter 5, page 117.)

Parents need as much time to talk when no reason can be found for their baby's death as when the reason is absolutely clear. The need to know 'why' is very strong, and if there is no explanation for their baby's death, it can be very hard for parents to accept it. Taking time to talk through what is known, and to understand what is not, can be helpful.

Even after a follow-up appointment, parents often find that questions and uncertainties continue to crop up. Some hospitals recognise this and encourage parents to return for more information or discussion if they need to do so. Some give the name and number of a contact person whom parents can visit or phone.

While they are in hospital, in the period immediately after their baby's death, parents also need information about what they might do for themselves and for their baby, and what others might do for them. There is much that parents can do to help themselves, and many ways in which positive memories can be created, but it is often hard for parents to think of these things for themselves. They need to know about the choices open to them, and they need information which will help them make those choices. Otherwise, there can be bitter regrets, as there were for Anne. She chose not to see her son, Philip, after he had died:

'The young doctor asked if we would like to see Philip, but we declined the offer — a decision I will regret to my dying day. If only someone could have talked to me, could have explained how important it was to say goodbye to our baby, could have told me how it would help with the grieving process, could have just gently taken me by the hand and supported me.'

There are many parents who feel that, at one point or another, they made a wrong decision, failed to do something or failed to ask that something should be done, and who are left saying 'if only'. Of course, there are bound to be some regrets: it is in the nature of bereavement to feel 'if only'. But if all parents were given the kind of information and support which Anne would have liked, a lot of unnecessary regrets could be avoided.

## Information parents need
After their baby's death, parents need information about:

- how, where and for how long their baby's body will be kept
- whom to ask if they wish to see their baby again
- what they might do for their baby (for example, washing and dressing their baby in special clothes, taking their baby's body home for a time, leaving a photo or special toy with their baby)
- mementos they could collect (for example, photographs, locks of hair, hand and foot prints, a cot card, stills from scans, fetal monitor tracing)
- religious ceremonies that can be carried out in hospital if they wish (a blessing or naming ceremony, for example)
- how their baby died and, if possible, why. (If there is no known reason for the death, parents need to know this.)
- the post-mortem (including what information a post-mortem might provide, and when and how they will receive the results; where, when and by whom the post-mortem will be carried out; when they will be able to see their baby again, if they wish to)
- implications for a future pregnancy
- how to suppress lactation
- contraception (if appropriate)

- registration, including the name of the registrar, address and office hours of the registry office, and the information that parents need to take there. (In the UK at present, there are no registration procedures for babies born dead before the legal age of viability.)
- funerals, burial and cremation (including information about the range of possible ceremonies, how these can be arranged, local facilities, and costs)
- services and sources of support (both professional and voluntary) available to them on leaving hospital
- what follow-up care they will receive (for example, the postnatal/follow-up appointment, home visits)
- whom to contact for further information after they have left hospital.

The way this information is communicated is just as important as the information itself. It is hard for parents to take in what is being said when they are upset and under stress. Often the information itself is upsetting or unfamiliar (information about a post-mortem or about funeral arrangements, for example). Parents need staff to be clear, honest and direct. The truth can hurt, but it is much more hurtful to feel that facts are being hidden or distorted. Parents need conversations which are unhurried and give them the time they need to clarify what they don't immediately understand. Often they need to be able to go back over the same information a second or even third time, perhaps on two or three different occasions. Above all, they need to feel at ease with the professional who is talking to them. It is difficult to accept information from a person who seems unsympathetic, unconcerned or embarrassed.

## TIME

What happens in hospital can happen very quickly and after their baby's death, many parents are left in a state of great shock and confusion, unable to grasp the truth of what has happened. They feel as though they have been dreaming or acting in a play. Afterwards they need time to catch up with reality.

Almost all parents need time with their baby's body. Not all want this straight away, but at some point most usually need to quietly hold and cuddle their baby, getting to know him or her and feeling close, before they have to say goodbye. Memories of this time can be the most precious that parents have. Naomi, whose daughter, Rosanna, died in her womb when she was eight and a half months pregnant, treasures the experience of being with her baby. She says, 'In a day — and a lifetime to come — of pain and loss, seeing Rosanna was the high point.'

Parents also need private time with each other; there is a particular need for privacy after a baby's death. Hospitals are very public places, and almost all bereaved parents have a pressing need to be somewhere secure and private. None want to feel isolated or abandoned, but most want to be away from other parents with live, healthy babies, somewhere where they can express their grief. So hospitals should provide a quiet, private, comfortable room where parents can stay and, if they wish, spend time with their baby; it is, after all, the only time that they have together. Many hospitals now provide, at the very least, a separate room, with a camp bed so that the baby's father can stay overnight. Some provide much more: a pleasant, specially decorated and comfortably furnished room, quite unlike a normal hospital room, with a double bed, a kettle, tea and coffee, and so on. There is a moses basket for the baby, and other members of the family are made welcome if the parents want them to be there. If a woman has no partner, then a relative or close friend is made just as welcome.

Parents need time to make decisions. They cannot feel clear about what is right for them and for their baby unless they have time to think and to talk. There is no reason why decisions about a funeral, for example, have to be made quickly, and every reason for making them slowly and with consideration. Sometimes some kind of time limit is helpful because an infinite amount of time can make decisions harder rather than easier to make, but this is no argument for rush or pressure. If decisions are rushed, there are often regrets later.

Finally, parents need time to talk with the professionals who have cared for them through their pregnancy and, most particularly, at the time of their baby's death. It can help to be able to go through exactly what happened, perhaps more than once, and to talk around it. By doing this, parents can begin to fix events in their minds, and feel that they have some grasp of what has happened. Often it is only hospital staff who can fulfil this role because only they have been fully involved in what has happened.

In 1991, the UK Stillbirth and Neonatal Death Society published guidelines for professionals on the management of miscarriage, stillbirth and neonatal death. These include detailed recommendations for the care of parents in hospital. The 'Principles of Good Practice' set out in the guidelines are reproduced on pages 235—41.

## HOSPITAL MANAGEMENT OF MISCARRIAGE*

The quality of care which parents receive in hospital is determined in part by hospital policy and in part by the resources available and the way those resources are used. Even more, however, the quality of care depends on the professionals who give that care, and not only on their skills but also on their understanding — their understanding of parents' needs and feelings, and of the meaning of a baby's death.

Both stillbirth and neonatal death are now much better understood, and the care parents receive in hospital has improved accordingly. Fifteen to twenty years ago it was common for parents' experiences to be minimised. It was unusual, for example, for parents to be given their stillborn baby to hold, and many did not even see their baby. Nowadays, the significance of a baby's death is recognised and parents are encouraged to hold and spend time with their baby.

But this understanding has not yet been fully extended to loss through miscarriage. Many parents who suffer a miscarriage find

*At the time of this book's publication, the age of viability in the UK is legally defined as twenty-eight weeks gestation. Babies born dead before twenty-eight weeks are regarded by the law as non-viable. They are said to have been miscarried, and they have no legal status. There is no legal requirement to register these earlier deaths, or to bury or cremate the body.

that their loss is regarded by professionals as a 'lesser' event than a stillbirth, and therefore as less upsetting. This may happen even when a miscarriage happens late in pregnancy, at a time when the baby might, if born alive, stand a chance (even if a very slim one) of survival. Ruby lost her baby at twenty-three weeks gestation:

> 'The nurse said, "It's better you lost it now. It would have been awful if you'd gone to term." I can't forgive her for saying that. How could she think it would comfort me? Faith was my baby.'

Yvonne came across the same lack of understanding when her daughter died at twenty-one weeks of pregnancy. The medical and legal terminology which the professionals used to describe her baby's death was not just irrelevant to her experience, it was also upsetting:

> 'I am confused as to what my baby is classed as. A bereavement officer called her an unviable fetus. My GP says she was a potential baby. But she is my baby, fully formed. I did not miscarry her, I had to go through an induced, very painful labour. I did not have her terminated. But because she was twenty-one weeks and not twenty-eight weeks, she was not a stillbirth. Lucy is my baby. How can anybody class her as anything else?'

Five years before she lost Lucy, Yvonne had lost another baby daughter, who was stillborn. So she has particular reason to know what little difference there really is between what is termed a 'miscarriage' and what a stillbirth.

For each parent, the loss of their baby has a very particular, personal meaning that has little to do with the timing of the loss. To suggest that it is less traumatic to lose a baby at, say, twenty-two weeks than at thirty-two, simply because the pregnancy has been ten weeks shorter, is to misunderstand how individual the experience of loss is. There is no scale of suffering which means that parents suffer more or differently depending on the point at which their baby dies. And there is no rule which says that the death of a baby who had a chance of life is more or less distressing than the death of a baby who could never have lived. Professionals, because they care for many parents, are able to compare one kind of loss with another. But to parents themselves, comparisons are meaningless. Parents know only what they have experienced: loss and grief cannot, and should not, be categorised.

Even so, miscarriage *is* still categorised by many professionals as a less significant loss, and hospital care often reflects this. Among all the hundreds of letters and accounts from parents which have been used in writing this book, those which describe poor hospital care are most often from parents whose baby 'miscarried'. Mary M, for example, began to lose amniotic fluid when she was just twenty-one weeks pregnant:

'I woke up one morning thinking at first that I had wet myself. I soon realised I hadn't, contacted the hospital and went in immediately. I was taken to the labour ward and examined. My husband was asked to wait outside but I feel I should have had him with me as I was very frightened. The midwife who prepared me for the examination did not have a pleasant manner and I took an immediate dislike to her. She asked me some questions which I couldn't really understand, and eventually I realised that she was implying that this could happen to women whose partners had treated them roughly during sexual intercourse. I was shocked and upset at this. The doctor then came in and examined me, and confirmed that it was liquor that I was losing and said in an offhand way, over his shoulder while he was doing something else, "Oh, you're miscarrying." I just felt devastated. They left me alone for some time until I reminded them that my husband was outside and could I see him. I was admitted that day and put on complete bed rest. The same doctor, when he came round, encouraged me to get up and walk around and leave it to fate.'

Rachel was twenty-three weeks pregnant when a scan showed that her baby had died. She was admitted to hospital straight away and her labour was induced. After the birth, she saw her baby briefly before the midwife took him (or her — Rachel never learnt the sex of her baby) away. Her husband did not see the baby, and they do not know what was done with the body. Afterwards, Rachel found it extremely difficult to accept her loss because it had been so minimised by the hospital:

'It was my first baby and I didn't know what to expect or what to ask for. I was too frightened and shocked to be able to argue or demand anything. I suppose I accepted the hospital's attitude, which was that what was happening to me was not important. Afterwards, this made me feel that the depression and sadness I felt must be abnormal.'

Fortunately, an increasing number of hospitals are now recognising the need to provide more sensitive care to women who miscarry; and some now make little distinction between the management of miscarriage and the management of stillbirth, treating parents with similar consideration. An increasing number of parents are now able to hold and spend time with their baby after a miscarriage, if they wish to do so, and with the help and support of hospital staff, they make their own choices about a funeral and either burial or cremation. The baby's body is treated as respectfully as any human body should be, and parents are encouraged to name their baby, talk about him or her, to bathe and dress the body if possible, and gather mementos. In some hospitals, all of this is usual practice, not only for babies who might have lived but also for babies who die at much earlier gestations.

Such improvements in the hospital management of miscarriage depend to some extent on the allocation of resources to this area of care, and to a large extent on professional training. In the end, practice will not improve until the professionals concerned (policy-makers as well as practitioners) have a better understanding of what miscarriage can mean, and are able to develop the skills they need to give appropriate care. Parents themselves can play an important part in bringing about change, working with professionals to promote better understanding of what the experience of miscarriage is like.

## PROFESSIONAL ATTITUDES

In the end, it is usually the people — the nurses, midwives, doctors and others — who matter most to parents in hospital. Even if the hospital is grim and institutional, if there's no privacy, no suitable accommodation and if the hospital routine gives way to no one's needs, just one understanding and caring person can transform parents' experience. Yvonne's midwife, Mary, was with her when a scan showed that her baby had died:

'Throughout the morning Mary stayed with me, comforting me, holding me. She spoke very gently and kindly, and showed so much care. I named the baby after her because she was so very kind to me that morning.

'After leaving hospital, I never expected to see her again, but one afternoon the door bell rang and when I opened the door, it was Mary. I felt so moved that she had taken the trouble to come and see me. We chatted over tea (well, I talked, she listened) and when it was time for her to leave she just touched my arm. It meant so much because I knew she understood how sad I was.'

Many parents are moved and greatly helped by the care which professionals give and the sympathy and understanding they show, not just at the time of a baby's death but also afterwards. They remember with gratitude the professionals who cried with them, who put out a hand or gave an embrace, who attended a funeral or memorial service, who sent flowers, wrote, phoned, or came to see them at home.

However, some parents find that their memories of their baby's death are made harder rather than easier to live with because of the attitudes of the professionals who cared for them. Sometimes there is a particular cause of distress, but most commonly it is the offhandedness of the professionals which upsets and offends parents, and an apparent lack of understanding, sympathy or concern.

Janet P's daughter, Emma, was cared for in hospital for a month and a half before she died. Throughout that time, Janet found it hard to build up a relationship with the special care baby unit staff:

'The doctor who had been present at delivery did talk to me regularly for the first two weeks but then suddenly disappeared for a fortnight. The nurses changed continually, and I hardly knew their names. Many did not wear badges or introduce themselves, and I wondered if they even knew which mum belonged to which baby. I desperately wanted to get to know them better. I wanted to feel more comfortable when visiting Emma, and I wanted them to like me so that they would look after my baby properly.

'I tried to be present for ward rounds but found that the doctors often did not acknowledge my presence. No one doctor seemed to be in charge of communicating with us and at times it was hard to find anyone to talk to . . .

'We were at home when the phone call came to tell us that Emma had died. We drove straight to the hospital but the porter had apparently not been told to expect us and asked why we had come. The nurse on duty was very sympathetic, but the doctor acted as if this sort of thing happened all the time. We would have found it easier if the staff had shown some emotion. We would have hoped that they did at least care something for her.

'We returned in the morning to deal with the paperwork and were told the post-mortem would be carried out within a couple of days and that we would then come back to discuss the results. In fact, the doctor phoned on the morning of the funeral to say that nothing positive had been discovered and that we should wait for further test results before seeing him. We never heard from him again.

'Apart from a visit by the social worker, no one from the unit contacted us. There were no flowers for Emma nor even a card, and no one attended the funeral. I would have liked someone who knew her to have come. We had always been told she had her own personality, yet no one seemed to notice that she had gone.'

There are many reasons why professionals fail to support parents. Some, of course, simply lack the imagination to feel what another person is feeling. Others do not understand because they themselves have not experienced anything which would help them to understand. They may never have been bereaved, for example, or may never have had or wanted children. And sometimes understanding is limited simply because of the way people are. Many people, for example, are frightened of drama and intense emotion: they cannot cope with it and try to avoid it or pretend it is not there.

Yet all professionals are saddened when a baby dies, some acutely so. All feel for the parents, and many share a little of the parents' grief. Sue, for example, a midwife, wrote this after caring for Jean and Chris, whose son, Ian, was stillborn:

'My own grief for Ian was insignificant compared to that of Jean and Chris, but it is important to realise that we, the care-givers, do have our own grief. I knew that I had to cry, and eventually, when watching a particularly sad television programme, the tears came. I left the room and sat on the kitchen floor and cried and cried and cried.'

It is right that professionals who are so closely involved with grieving parents should also grieve themselves. But some find it hard to control what they are feeling, or to express it in the right way. This may be because they are reminded of their own experiences of loss, or perhaps because they feel unsupported in their work and are under stress. Some, perhaps because of lack of experience or lack of training, or both, simply cannot set aside their own painful feelings sufficiently to be able to help and support parents.

At a professional level, nurses, midwives and doctors may see a baby's death as a failure. They may feel responsible and blame themselves, even though there may be no reason for blame. They may also feel inadequate and helpless. Most want to offer comfort, but they are also very aware that they are powerless to provide what parents most want and need: they simply cannot bring back the pregnancy that has ended or the baby who has died.

These reasons are not excuses. Nothing can excuse poor care or uncaring attitudes at a time of such need. But clearly, professionals have a difficult job to do, and if they are to be enabled to do that job well, their own needs must also be met. Fundamentally, there is a need for adequate professional training: professionals cannot be expected to understand the needs of parents unless they have been able to learn what those needs are; nor can they be expected to provide proper care unless they are equipped with relevant knowledge and skills. Equally important, professionals need to work within appropriate operational policies; they need to feel confident that not just their own personal practice but the system as a whole is sensitive to parents' needs. Each hospital and each health authority should have a clear and detailed policy for the management of miscarriage, stillbirth and neonatal death, and this policy should be shared and understood by all the staff involved. Finally, if professionals are to provide parents with the quality of care that they need, it is essential that they themselves have access to support. They too need opportunities to share problems or talk about their feelings.

## GOING BACK: LATER CONTACT WITH THE HOSPITAL

For many parents, the hospital is the only home their baby ever had and the only place where they were ever together as a family.

Returning home, with no baby and so few memories, they can feel as though what happened in the hospital — even their baby — was a dream. Linda B's baby, James, died in her womb when she was just over seven months pregnant. This is how she describes the day she and her husband, Paul, left hospital:

> 'I got dressed and we waited around until we were told that we could go. While we were waiting, we talked a bit more and then I cried a lot more. Now it was becoming all too real. While we were in hospital, it didn't seem too bad — we could shut the whole world out. But once we left, we knew we'd have to face everybody. We both didn't really want to leave. We just wanted to stay in that room for ever and ever.'

Laura had similar feelings when she left hospital after the birth of her twins, Hannah and Katie. Hannah survived after a period in special care; Katie died an hour after she was born. Laura had had close contact with the hospital from the time that it became known that Katie could not survive:

> 'After we found out in the twenty-fourth week of my pregnancy that Katie would not survive, I needed — and had — an awful lot of support from the hospital team. This continued through the rest of my pregnancy (which was stressful and complicated), during the birth and in the days after Katie's death. I grew to trust the staff and felt very safe in their care. When it was time for me to leave hospital, I knew my care would be handed over to the community team, but for me this felt inappropriate. I wanted to continue to share my feelings with the people who had come to know me over the months, and who had known both Katie and Hannah. For some time afterwards, I especially wanted to go and talk to the midwives who had seen Katie, to recount the birth and the time we had with her. It was as if I needed Katie's short life to be given recognition, and confirmation that the aching love I felt belonged to someone who had really existed.'

There are, of course, some parents who do not want to go near the hospital where they lost their baby, and know that it would not help them to do so. But for parents like Laura (including parents whose babies did not live after birth), it can help to have some continued contact with the hospital, to go back and talk with the people who knew their baby, or to go back and simply be there, just for a short while. Doing this can confirm that what happened was real, and can bring back the memories which, however painful, all parents need. It can be a way of grieving, and many feel better after doing it. For Sue R it was certainly helpful:

'As I was having problems coping with Naomi's death, I asked if I could see the hospital chaplain about two months later. He readily agreed and was most helpful. I saw him a few times and during my subsequent pregnancy. Although he had not experienced the death of a baby first hand, his counsel was invaluable. As he had met so many other grieving parents, he was able to tell me with authority that my reactions and emotions were normal. He was very prepared to spend time with me even some months after the event, when I was beginning to feel I should have got over it all. He also arranged for us to return to the hospital about three months after Naomi's birth. We were warmly received by the sister who had cared for us, given tea and were able to discuss Naomi and what had happened. We were shown the room where she was born. Our daughter, Lois, came with us and she was shown some newborn babies and thoroughly enjoyed seeing where *she* was born. It helped me to overcome my fear of returning to the hospital for any subsequent delivery, and the attitude of the staff was most healing to me.'

Some hospitals, recognising how devastated, isolated and lost parents can feel when they go home without their baby, make arrangements to keep in touch with parents and offer some continuing support. Many encourage parents to return to the hospital, although this is more common when a baby has spent a period in special care and less common if the baby has died before or immediately after birth. Some organise one or a series of home visits by medical or nursing staff, or a counsellor. This way, some links with the hospital are maintained, at least through the initial lonely time at home.

Louise had a different reason for returning to the hospital where her daughter died. She felt that she had been very sensitively cared for and wanted to commend the hospital for that, but both she and her husband also felt that they needed to ensure that other parents would not have to suffer, as they had, the agonising effects of faulty monitoring equipment:

'After lengthy, positive discussions with the consultant, we arranged to see the unit general manager of the hospital. Ready for an argument, we were pleasantly surprised at how understanding and conciliatory she was, acknowledging the poor service her unit had given us. Yes, she admitted, the machines were long overdue for replacement. She had already put in hand a review of the monitoring equipment and one new monitor had been purchased immediately and was in use as a direct result of our complaint. This meant a tremendous amount to us. We felt a great strength from the knowledge that our complaint had brought about such positive changes.'

In time, some parents develop new and different links with their hospital. Perhaps alone, or more usually along with other parents, they work in a number of ways to bring about improvements in both the standard of care and the hospital facilities. For Penny and her partner, fund-raising was important:

'Since Nicholas's death we have found that fund-raising for the special care unit at the hospital where he spent his entire life, has helped enormously. We definitely felt a need to stay in contact with the hospital as the doctors and nurses had been as much a "family" to Nicholas, as we had been. We also felt that this would give us something positive to focus on, so that his short life would not have been completely in vain.'

Rosalind found that returning to the hospital where her daughter died was difficult but also a very positive thing to do. Her own experience of hospital care had been good, and she felt she should do something to ensure that other parents were similarly well treated:

'The more I talk to other people, the more I realise that my experiences in hospital were unusual and many people don't get the right treatment, so I was keen to talk to midwives and doctors. I went back to the hospital recently and spoke to a group and will do so again in future. It is very difficult, but if it helps someone else then it starts not to make sense of Georgia's death but to make it more positive, and in doing so gives her more dignity.'

Many parents feel a need to create something positive out of the negative experience of their baby's death. Since the hospital is usually such an important place in their memories, and is for many the backdrop to all their memories of their baby's life and death, returning there in a more positive role can be helpful, and an important way of remembering and commemorating their baby.

# 4  Grief and Grieving

Grief is very private and often very lonely. Only the grieving person fully understands what they have lost and what this means to them, and it is difficult, and sometimes impossible, for them to describe their feelings of loss to others. Even those who are very close to them may not be able to understand or share in their grief.

Because grief is so isolating, most of us know little about what profound grief is like until we experience it ourselves. As a result, the experience can be bewildering and sometimes frightening. Most bereaved parents, at some time, wonder whether their thoughts and feelings are 'normal', and whether their sadness will ever become bearable. This chapter describes what grief is like for parents who have lost a baby. We look at ways of grieving, of finding support when it is needed and, eventually, of easing the pain.

## FEELINGS OF GRIEF

'I just want things to be normal again, I want the hole inside me to fill up, I want to sleep at night without sobbing my heart out, most of all I want my baby. I scream inside for her. I want a lot, don't I? Some I can have, one I never will.'

After their baby's death, parents grieve for the baby they have lost, and for all that their baby meant to them. They also grieve for a lost future — their baby's future, their own future as their baby's parents, and the future they would have shared as a family. They grieve because they have lost an expected happiness. Many feel that they have also lost hope.

Grief is, for everyone, this acute, overwhelming sense of loss, a feeling of emptiness and a great longing for what has been taken away. Parents long for their baby to hold, to cuddle, to feed, to care for, and, most of all, to love. It can be difficult to believe that such intense longing will never be fulfilled and that what is wanted and needed so much can never be had. Coming to grasp the permanence of loss is very hard, and once grasped, it is very painful.

Along with the pain and sadness, grief brings other feelings which may come and go, change and change again, over a long period of time. There is often guilt, anger, bitterness or resentment; feelings of helplessness, loneliness, or the futility of living; great anxiety, fear and sometimes panic. There are almost always physical effects too. Not surprisingly, bereaved people often feel physically exhausted — yet they may be unable to rest or sleep. Many feel listless and without energy. Some find they become short of breath, suffer tightness in the throat or chest, or feel they are suffocating. There can be unexplained headaches or other aches and pains, stomach upsets or diarrhoea. Some parents say that their arms ache for the baby they cannot hold.

Many parents who lose a baby have never been bereaved before and have never had to grieve. Many are shocked by the intensity of what they feel — and may continue to feel over months and maybe years. Initially, their shock may be all the greater because of the suddenness with which they are cut off from the future they had imagined and looked forward to:

'Last year I became the happiest person on earth when I found out I was pregnant. But today I feel lost, I don't feel worthy of living, I feel a failure and I don't know where I'm heading any more.'

Many bereaved parents feel that nothing is important any more, that life — their own life in particular — has lost its meaning and purpose. After his son, Jonathon, was stillborn, Tim felt there was only one thing which he wanted and which mattered — yet he could not have it:

'My boss wanted to know why I wasn't giving work 100 per cent. His view was that the job should always come first. I felt nothing came first any more. There was no longer any point running for buses or queuing in shops — everything became unimportant in comparison to the desire to have our baby back.'

Many parents also suffer a complete loss of confidence in themselves. They felt helpless in the face of their baby's death because they were unable to prevent it, and the feelings of helplessness continue afterwards and become feelings of worthlessness and failure. Some parents feel very strongly that they *should* have been able, as so many other parents are able, to have a live, healthy baby, and they feel that their baby's death is, if not their fault, certainly their failure. Many parents punish themselves with these feelings:

> 'Like many others, I lost all sense of worth, felt useless and had no confidence in anything I did. Most of all, I now know, I never felt worthy of giving myself any praise. I felt a failure, and I tried to carry on as normal to compensate for failing everyone else.'

Many parents feel that they have not just failed their baby and themselves, but they have also let down their partner, perhaps other children, and the rest of their family. Often they feel that they add to these failures by showing their misery, crying, by being unable to put on a calm or cheerful face or being what they see as 'weak' or not coping. Unfortunately, this can mean that they hold in and hide their grief, and this in turn can make it harder to bear.

For Jane, feelings of failure were acute. Her daughter, Jemma, died in her womb when she was thirty-eight weeks pregnant. No reason was ever found. Jane was 31 years old, and until this tragedy happened, neither she nor her husband had experienced any kind of catastrophe or anything that felt like failure. She had been successful at school as a child, had done well in exams, qualified as a teacher and started a career. She was thrilled to conceive in the month that she had planned, went on teaching until she was six months pregnant, moved house at eight months, and felt on top of the world. There had been no problems at all. So, two months after Jemma's death, Jane found herself 'mentally on a precipice':

> 'Miraculously, I have a teaching job on a term's basis. I start next week. But the prospect terrifies me. I am afraid of most things now. I have no desire to sort out the house, can only force myself to cook and don't really eat anything. The mornings are the worst. This morning my

nerves were so bad I was violently sick several times.

'I am so desperate to try and resume a happy life for my husband's sake, and so afraid I can't ever recover, as I truly do often feel I would prefer to die. I never knew there was such suffering in the world before. I have always been so lucky and happy, and now I just cannot see a way ahead without my daughter. I have no faith whatsoever in a God now, nor does my husband. I truly don't see how anyone can have when they've held their own dead baby. There is no meaning whatsoever in such pain.'

For a long time, Jane saw what had happened to her, and her misery, as some kind of wrongdoing on her part, and her feelings of failure, and of responsibility for what had happened, made it hard for her to grieve:

'I still see it as my "crime" within the family. I don't talk to them about it because I feel I mustn't bring up all the pain for them again. I did so much damage at the time. Having a grave is just my permanent punishment for what I did. (I feel guilty saying this because Jemma wouldn't want to have caused such pain.)'

Feelings of guilt cause a lot of pain and sometimes take years to resolve. But six years after Jemma's death, Jane was able to write:

'For the days around the anniversary of Jemma's death, and her birth ten days later, all the pain comes flooding back, and I know it will always be that way. But day to day, she is now peaceful and safe inside. I carry her always. She is wholly mine, my private sadness but also my perfect, secret joy.'

Parents often feel to blame for their baby's death, particularly, perhaps, when no satisfactory medical explanation is given or can be found. Since it is natural to feel that there *must* be a reason for a baby's death, the absence of any medical explanation often leaves parents with the feeling that they themselves were in some way responsible:

'I am furious that no one has asked me questions to prove to them and me that I didn't do anything. I *badly* want answers to *how* these things happen. I feel a totally unresolved confusion about how a perfect baby, on the end of a perfect (or so they told me) placenta, in a perfectly healthy mother, can possibly be lost. I feel I did it.'

Some parents do not blame themselves but still feel angry or bitter because there seems to have been no reason for their baby to die. Many feel, simply and strongly, that what has happened should not have happened. Many feel that it should not have happened *to them*. Kim's son was born prematurely after Kim caught a kidney and bladder infection:

> 'There are mothers who drink, smoke and take drugs in their pregnancies but they still have healthy babies that survive. Then there are women like me. I didn't smoke, drink or take drugs in my pregnancy, I watched my diet and I took care of myself, and look what happened. Life's just so unfair.'

In one way or another, almost all parents compare themselves with others, and inevitably feel jealous of those who have successful pregnancies and live, healthy babies. Many find it hard to admit their jealousy, although it is natural and understandable, and this adds to their sense of isolation. Their experience of tragedy seems to cut them off from friends and acquaintances whose experiences are so much happier. Pat describes her feelings of jealousy after she lost her twins:

> 'I feel terribly jealous of two women, and sometimes the feelings are very strong. The first gave birth to baby twin girls a week before our twins were born. Every time I see her with her double pushchair I feel very upset, then very jealous of her, which I suppose is understandable really. The other woman had a baby boy two months premature. He was not expected to live. I felt sorry for the family, whom I know quite well, but at the same time I was strangely pleased that we would have something in common. However, against all the odds, the baby has recovered and now I feel terribly jealous of her and I feel so guilty about it. It seems so unfair that my perfectly-formed babies died, and hers lived.'

Jealousy is a part of the wanting which all parents feel after their baby's death. This wanting can continue for a long time, often for years, for the simple reason that it can never be fulfilled. The baby who has died can never be brought back, can never be replaced. Sallie's first baby, James, died when he was ten days old. Ten years later, Sallie still misses him and has come to realise that she will always do so:

'Friends forget, of course they do. Only a few remember with you. But you yourself need to go on remembering. I still miss James and I know that it will always be like this. I still feel envy, plain and simple, when other women become pregnant. When it's friends, I'm genuinely glad, but I can't help the envy. It's worse with people I don't know.'

Feelings of grief do not necessarily disappear as the years go by. Time may change them and almost always makes them more bearable: most parents say, years after their baby's death, that the passing of time has helped. They also say that the memory of their baby never fades, and that there are at least some feelings which they know will remain with them always. It is, as one father describes it, 'a necessary sadness'.

## REMINDERS

There are moments in everyone's grieving which are particularly painful because something happens, or is said, which brings all the feelings of sadness and despair to the surface. This happens often during the first year or so after the death, but even many years later, often quite unpredictably, wounds can be opened up again and the pain of early grief comes flooding back:

'. . . it may be seeing a little boy on the beach playing with his daddy, or seeing a pram the same colour as the one we wanted, or hearing a mother shout "Christopher". We never know what is going to trigger off the water works.'

Throughout the year, certain dates and events inevitably bring back memories of both happiness and tragedy. Jean had celebrated her birthday the previous year with special happiness, because her pregnancy had just been confirmed:

'This year my birthday would have been a sad enough day in any case, because neither of us felt up to celebrating. But also I couldn't help but remember what I'd been thinking and feeling on the same day only a year before. I was so excited then, so pleased with myself. It makes me think now what a fool I was. I can hardly believe that, at that time, I really did expect everything to be happy ever after.'

For parents whose babies were born prematurely, the date when their baby would have been due can be a difficult hurdle. The day is a clear reminder of 'what should have been', and often this is underlined by the birth of other babies due at the same time. Lyn's daughter, Amy, was stillborn when Lyn was thirty-four weeks pregnant, and two months later Lyn faced a particularly difficult time:

> 'This week has been very hard for me. The women who were due at about the same time as me have all had their babies and I seem to run into them at every corner. I had three people in one day ask me what I had and then almost shrivel up. I don't know who felt worse, them or me. Then, through the post yesterday I received my free bag of baby samples. I must have cried for two hours solid, just sitting in the chair, rocking back and forth, hugging a disposable nappy to my chest.'

For Christina, it was the birth of her sister's baby that brought her loss home to her:

> 'My sister had a little girl three weeks after me and although I took it OK and I held her and felt all right, it hit me a few days after and I was really bad, so distraught. I went numb and couldn't stop crying loudly and I was shaking and my teeth were chattering. I thought it was a nervous breakdown.'

The birth of other babies, whether to others in the family or to friends, is always difficult for bereaved parents to cope with and is always likely to revive their grief, even years after their baby's death. In the same way, parents often feel saddened when they come into contact with children of about the same age as their baby would have been, had he or she lived:

> 'I saw a lady today who had a little girl just after I had Suzanne, and she was bouncing her around, laughing and kissing her. It hurt so much. It just made me think how Suzanne would now have been a lovely age (nearly 7 months), and how we would have been enjoying the sunshine together.'

Although all parents continue to think about the baby they have lost as a baby, some also think of their baby as a growing child. As the years go by, they think about what their baby would now look like or would now be doing, if he or she had lived. Inevitably, seeing other children of about the right age reminds parents of what might have been. Peter's son, John, was born two and a half years after his brother James died. When John found a friend just over two years older than himself, Peter found it sad to see the two boys together: 'I look at them and think, this is how it should have been.' Many parents live with the feeling that their family is incomplete because one child is, and always will be, missing. Many find it hard to know what to answer when people ask them how many children they have.

This feeling of incompleteness can be very strong when a twin baby dies. There are not just occasional but constant reminders of the baby who has died. Gail gave birth to twin daughters. Julie was stillborn; Eleanor was alive and healthy:

> 'The thing I always remember people saying, not to us but about us, was "Well, at least they have one baby." Oh yes, I agree, and for that we are very lucky. But we also have a constant reminder of what should have been. Every time Eleanor does something for the first time, it should be a happy moment. But it isn't, it's a mixed-up, emotional moment. Her first birthday was terrible. I cried nearly all day and then felt guilty. Then when I did manage to smile and be happy, I felt guilty again.'

For many parents, the anniversaries of their baby's birth and death are extremely hard. Even years later, parents can find that on those days their grief is almost as painful as it was in the beginning, and many approach the day with real dread, not knowing how or whether they will be able to cope. In the same way, any special day or family occasion — birthdays, Christmas, Mother's and Father's Day — can bring thoughts and feelings about the baby to the surface and can be hard to deal with.

But sometimes it can also be a relief to think about and cry for the baby. After the first weeks and months, grief so often has to be put aside in order to be able to carry on with day-to-day living. Some parents come to feel that they actually need occasions when they can give special time to the baby they have lost, and when they can express what they felt and still feel for him or her. In particular, although anniversaries are so sad and difficult, they can become special days:

'The day of Simon's birthday is also the day that he died. It is a day that I have always wanted to commemorate, even celebrate somehow. Rituals have become important to me, as is reliving and talking through the events of that day and the days leading up to it. The rituals involve allowing myself "time out" on this very special day to spend as I feel best reflects my particular mood. In all but one year I have taken the day off work in order to visit the crematorium where our entry was made in the book of remembrance. Much time is spent also looking through "Simon's Book", a collection of treasured items, for instance, photos of a pregnant me, co-op card, kick chart, cot tag, birth certificate, bereavement cards, death certificate, etc.'

Grief is always difficult and painful but, so long as it is given some course to run, it need not be destructive. 'Bad days', whether expected or unexpected, are certainly bad, but they are also opportunities to grieve, and without such opportunities, grief cannot progress. For many parents, these bad times have proved to be turning points in the progress of their grief.

## OBSTACLES TO GRIEVING

Grieving is the experience and expression of grief. It is both necessary and healing. But there is much that can get in its way and make it hard. Often there are obstacles which have to be overcome before parents can grieve as they need to. The biggest obstacle of all, especially at first, is that grieving is simply too painful:

'Sometimes I try to block it out that I was ever pregnant, because when I try to come to terms with it, it breaks my heart.'

But it is not only fear of heartbreak which prevents parents grieving. Sometimes it can seem selfish to grieve. Diane, like many parents, felt she should hold back from expressing her grief for the sake of her husband and her two older daughters:

'I had to be strong for my husband and children. I held all my pain in and just lived each day as it came. I tried to pretend it hadn't happened.'

Often it is the baby's father who feels he must be strong and who sets his own grief aside. Conventionally, men are expected to take on a supportive role and to show their feelings less. As a result, a father's grief can go unrecognised:

'My husband was never really thought of during the weeks following our son's death. Friends always asked him how *I* was and I even had several bouquets addressed solely to me. He suffered greatly.'

Tim felt that, as a man, he was not allowed to express his grief as he needed to:

'Fathers are just as upset as mothers when a baby dies. They get involved, they feel the baby growing in its mother's stomach, feel it kicking. It's their child too. Yet men are supposed to be able to get on with things. We aren't supposed to sit at our desks and cry. Other men may come up and say "If you need to talk, I'm here," but they don't mean it. Men don't like listening to other men's problems.'

Many parents — both men and women — find that other people do not acknowledge the importance and significance of their baby's death and do not understand their need to grieve. This can lead them to suppress their grief, feeling either that they should not feel as they do, or that they must not upset or embarrass others by showing it. Five months after her son, Daniel, was stillborn, Juanita wrote:

'I get days when all I want to do is cry, but I feel I am upsetting everyone else. Although my husband and I talk about Daniel nearly every day, he isn't mentioned by anyone else. My parents, my in-laws, brother and sister haven't mentioned the baby since it happened. They ask me how I am occasionally but that is all. I feel that it has been passed over like a visit to the dentist.'

Celia, who lost one twin, felt similarly let down by her family and friends:

'They tried to understand and were certainly very kind to me in the early weeks. But they all expected me to be "over it" very quickly, especially because they felt I'd got one baby (the surviving twin) and they felt this made it less bad for me.'

Linda S also suffered because the significance of her baby's death was overlooked, not just by her family and friends but by hospital staff. After experiencing very poor hospital care, Linda was left with very few memories and mementos and with a great many regrets, which made it difficult for her to grieve:

> 'They asked me if I wanted to see the baby, but at the time I was so drugged up and so tired I just said no. Now I wish I had seen her. We both feel we would have had something to grieve over. As it is, it sometimes seems as if it never happened to us. If they had given us a few days and then asked if we wanted to see our baby and bury our baby, it would have been different. I wish we had buried her and had a photo of her, not to stare at all the time but to look at now and then, just so I know there was something there.'

It is perhaps more likely that a baby's death will be minimised and misunderstood when it happens relatively early in pregnancy. Parents may be told that they are 'lucky' to have lost their baby when they did, and they may find that the death of their loved and wanted baby is regarded by others as a minor loss.

The lack of understanding some parents experience when their baby dies as a result of abnormalities can be equally hurtful. Often people, including professionals, fail to understand that the reason for a baby's death, or the baby's appearance, does not necessarily have any bearing on how parents feel, nor lessen in any way their need to grieve. In fact, the need to grieve may be greater. Callie's baby, Alan, died of thanatophoric dysplasia — a condition in which the baby is born with shortened limbs and often a large head. Callie suffered a great deal from other people's reactions to her son's death:

> 'The hardest part of Alan's death was the cruel remarks people made. Many's the time people have asked me how deformed he was. But to me, he was the most lovely child I ever saw. People also seem to think you should not mourn an abnormal baby. Why not? You carried it for nine months, it was part of you.'

Everyone needs recognition of their loss and of the cause of their sadness. It is extremely difficult to grieve for a baby whom others do not recognise, or to deal with feelings which others seem to think are unnecessary or inappropriate. All bereaved parents need to know that no matter why, when or how it happens, a baby's death is an event of immense significance and that grieving for their baby is necessary and right.

## COMING TO UNDERSTAND THE DEATH

It is hard to grasp the reality of any death, but the death of a baby is particularly hard to accept. It is so contrary to the natural order of things, usually so totally unexpected, so little spoken about and recognised, that it can seem utterly beyond comprehension. Yet coming to grasp the reality and finality of what has happened is a first step in grieving. Parents need to believe what seems so unbelievable, and somehow fit it into the pattern of their lives.

For most parents, this process of taking in the death begins with questions. Why did this happen? What went wrong? Was it something we did? Could it have been prevented? Could it happen again? After Fiona's third baby died, she urgently needed to know the reason:

> 'I think that's the most difficult thing, if you don't know why. You can come to terms with things if you know why. All I could see by then was that there had to be a reason for three babies to die.'

Eventually it was discovered that Fiona had lupus — a disease in which the body's immune system attacks the body's own tissues and organs. Although this was bad news, it was also a relief:

> 'When we had the reason, it was the most enormous relief. I know it seems odd, because we didn't have any babies, but at least we knew why. Just knowing, even though it may not change anything, makes it more bearable.'

Two years after the death of her daughter, Jemma, Jane's grief was still mainly focused on the need to understand *why*:

> 'Although on the face of it I have learnt to live with not having Jemma with us, and more importantly with the fact that she can't have her life, I still spend an awful lot of time thinking and thinking about what happened at the time and about her and what she would be like now, and so on. I do all my normal "tasks" perfectly well. I wouldn't even

say I was depressed. But I spend all my day-dreaming time just twisting it over and over. It's still normally the first thing I think of when I wake up, and I'm especially indulgent on long car journeys . . . I still feel that slightly suffocated feeling that no matter where I look and how hard I chew it over, I still can't find a reason or a compensatory thought. There still seems to have been no reason, no purpose, and I can't seem to fit it into my life as a meaningful episode at all.'

In their search for a reason, parents are likely to need answers to many different questions, but usually their first and most pressing need is to understand the medical events leading up to their baby's death and, if possible, what exactly the cause was. Many consent to a post-mortem examination of their baby in the hope that a definite cause of death will be revealed.

For some parents, these hopes are fulfilled and the post-mortem does provide a reason for their baby's death. But other parents are disappointed: sometimes the post-mortem is inconclusive, providing information which would not otherwise have been known but which still does not wholly explain the death; sometimes it gives no indication at all of why the baby died. And although some parents find it a comfort to discover that there was nothing wrong with their baby, Susan voices a response that is probably more common:

'The post-mortem revealed nothing. They said he was perfectly formed and there was nothing that could have made him die. I wished they had found a reason, just so I could come to terms with the fact that although he was perfect, there was a reason why he died. But there is nothing I can do to ease the pain I feel, knowing that although he was perfect, and we both loved and wanted him, he was still taken from us.'

Whether or not a cause is found for their baby's death, it is essential that parents are given all the information which is available, as well as opportunities to talk to the doctors concerned and ask questions. Even if it is impossible for doctors to give the clear and detailed explanation which parents want, it is always possible for them to share what *is* known with parents, and also to explain what is not known or not understood.

Unfortunately, this sharing of information does not always take place. Some parents are not given adequate information or time for discussion. Some are given information at a time when it is difficult for them to listen to — let alone discuss — the details of their baby's death. Later, they may find that they are unsure of what was said, or that they need to ask more questions to be able to understand it better. Ann was told that her baby had died because of placental insufficiency, yet she needed to know and understand much more:

'I am still left with so many questions. Why was this never noticed at any of my check-ups? Why were my blood pressure and urine always fine? Why did he not slow down in movement enough for the hospital to be concerned? He had always, up until it was too late, kicked more than ten times a day. Why did I not go into early labour when things started to go wrong? I will carry on always asking myself questions and wondering whether there was something I should have noticed.'

These are the sort of questions which parents need to be able to put to professionals and to which they need an honest response. It may be that there are no satisfactory answers, but it is easier for parents to live with this if professionals show that they understand the importance and legitimacy of parents' concerns, and are available for discussion as and when it is needed.

If parents feel, even years after their baby's death, that they need more information, then it is worth attempting to obtain it. If they feel they have questions still to ask, then it is worth asking them. There are several sources of information which parents can use. The hospital consultant (or consultants) concerned is likely to be able to provide the most detailed information. (We say more about obtaining information from the hospital on pages 117–8.) An appointment with the GP can also be helpful. After a baby's death, the hospital should pass on information to the parents' GP, including details of the post-mortem results, if one has been carried out. So the GP should be equipped to answer questions, and should certainly be prepared to talk. The community midwife and the health visitor may also be able to help and give time for discussion.

When making an appointment to see any of these professionals, it is wise to say why the appointment is wanted and why it would be valuable. The professional concerned should then be able to read through the medical notes (if available) beforehand, be better prepared, and allow enough time.

However not all professionals are sympathetic or willing to talk at length, and not all can communicate clearly. Some parents find that they have to look for information elsewhere. Many of the voluntary organisations listed on pages 245–8 offer both support and information to parents. Many specialise in offering support to parents whose babies have or have had specific conditions or abnormalities. Many have access to professional and expert advisers to whom they can sometimes refer inquiries.

But finding a medical explanation for a baby's death is only a part of most parents' search for a reason. There are usually other questions too, which may only surface once the medical cause has — or has not — been found. When Sandra was told that no medical cause could be found for her daughter's death, a new layer of questions emerged:

> 'We were told the results of the post-mortem and it showed my baby was perfect in every way, which made me feel more heartbroken, because if there was nothing wrong, why did she have to die? I remember saying, why me, why my baby, what had I done to deserve this?'

Even those parents who do receive an explanation for their baby's death may find that knowing the medical cause is not the same as understanding why their baby died. Answers to some questions can uncover other questions, to which there may be no answers at all. June was told that her son probably died because of an infection she contracted in pregnancy, but she realised that this information did not really 'explain' Philip's death:

> 'Even if you have logical answers, they don't address the real why. Why me? Why now? Why this innocent babe? We were endlessly reassured that it wasn't our fault, but although, after long grief-stricken months, I have come to accept what happened, to take renewed interest in myself and my career, even to understand how much good came out of the tragedy, I think the search for the answer to that why — the search for the very meaning of life — is a lifetime's work.'

Some parents are eventually able to find a meaning in their baby's death. For others, there comes a time when they feel they have to put their questions aside and try to accept that for them there will be no satisfactory answers or explanations. Most reach a stage when they are able to say that they understand as much as they are able to understand — and accept what has happened as far as it is possible to accept it. It is a compromise — but reaching that compromise is an important achievement.

## FUNERALS AND OTHER CEREMONIES

A funeral or ceremony of some kind can give parents an opportunity to express their grief and also their love for their baby. It can be a way of acknowledging a baby's importance, and it can create memories to hold onto in the future. It may also help parents to accept the reality of their loss. Parents often say that it was only at the funeral, when they saw their baby's tiny coffin, that they properly understood that their baby had died. Although this means that a funeral is distressing, it also makes it an important step forward:

> 'No one warned me that Sarah's coffin would be so small. Funerals always mean big cars, big coffins, not a shoe box. I think that was the hardest few hours. While I was in labour, I felt they could still be wrong. After, I thought I would wake up from this nightmare. Saying goodbye, that final goodbye, will always be such a vivid, sad memory.'

Although a funeral is generally thought of in traditional ways, it can, in fact, be adapted according to parents' wishes. For example, although a religious service is important for some parents and gives them some comfort, a funeral does not have to be a religious ceremony. It is important that parents are able to have the kind of funeral that they feel is right for them and their baby.

For Neil and Ita, holding a funeral for their son, Cian, helped not only them but also their two older children, Sam and Orla, aged 5 and 3, towards acceptance of Cian's death. Twelve days after he was born, Cian was found to have Edwards' syndrome (a fatal condition caused by a chromosome abnormality), and Neil

and Ita were told that he would not live long. They decided to
bring Cian home, and they were able to live together as a family
for three and a half weeks. During these weeks, the family
thought about Cian's approaching death and how they would say
goodbye. Neil and Ita visited the local cemetery and crematorium
with their other children:

> 'Responding to Sam and Orla's questions on that bright afternoon,
> we told them that when someone dies and their body doesn't work
> any more, you can't keep it because it would go bad and you can't
> just throw it away. "So you can do two things," we said. "You can
> put it on a special fire that turns the body into a special smoke which
> goes up the chimney and mixes with the air, or you can out it into
> the ground so that it mixes with the earth and helps flowers to grow.
> Which do you think would be best: mixing with the air, or with the
> earth?" Their reply was as matter-of-fact as if we'd asked them
> whether they wanted bread or toast for their tea: "With the earth." '

The family decided that Cian would be buried in a small babies'
section of the local cemetery and, with the agreement of family
and friends, that only Neil, Ita and the two children would be
there. Neil remembers:

> 'It was a spring-like day. We drove to a local flower shop and the four
> of us each selected flowers to place on Cian's grave. Then we collected
> Cian from the funeral home and drove to the cemetery with Ita and
> the children holding the coffin on their laps. Our two chosen priests —
> Catholic and Anglican — were waiting for us. We lowered Cian's
> coffin into the grave and the priests conducted a ceremony lasting
> only about five minutes. We finished by singing "All Things Bright
> and Beautiful". Then the grave was filled in and we were left in the
> warm sunshine to tidy it at our leisure. Ita and I cried quietly, the
> children played and then we took photographs. It was a sad but lovely
> day.'

For Tom and Rosalind, the funeral that they held for their
daughter, Georgia, did not meet all their needs. So, after the
funeral and cremation, they took some time to decide what else
they should do. They eventually decided to bury Georgia's ashes
at a place where they had spent a happy weekend before her birth.
They asked permission to bury her ashes there and to plant a tree,
with a plaque in her memory:

'We bought the tree and it was planted on a small hillock near a pond by a daffodil bank. The plaque reads simply "Georgia's tree", giving her full name and the date of her birth and death. We return there once or twice a year and visit the tree. Sometimes we plant bulbs, sometimes wild flowers, but always something. We take pictures of the tree, and of ourselves and the children around it. As the years roll by, I find each visit more easy to make, and I look forward to going. I look forward to having special time to concentrate on Georgia and tend the tree. The tree is also very special to all the children, even the two who were not born at the time of Georgia's death. The tree, to them, represents the sister they never knew, the funeral they never attended, and is how Georgia can somehow share their lives and they hers.'

Many parents do not have a grave or any kind of memorial to visit and lack a focus for their grief. Many (especially those whose babies died some years ago) did not hold a funeral. Some parents, who left arrangements after their baby's death to the hospital, do not know what happened to their baby's body and over the years that follow, may find this increasingly hard to live with. Many have a feeling of 'unfinished business'. They feel that they should have marked their baby's life and death in some way and made a proper ending to their experience. Not having done so, they find they can neither grieve as they want to grieve, nor allow their grief to rest.

Often it is possible, even many years after a baby's death, to make up for these omissions. It may, for example, be possible to locate where a baby is buried. Norma, whose son was stillborn, wrote to the hospital twelve years after his death to try to find out what had been done with his body:

'It has always been on my mind about my baby, not having anywhere to go and take flowers on his birthday or any time. After trying many times to write letters to see if I could find anything out, I finally succeeded. I phoned the maternity records department at the hospital and they gave me all the information about his birth and where he was buried. They told me to phone the cemetery. This I did, and within fifteen minutes I received a phone call from them giving me the details of his grave number and plot.

'Although it is a public grave, he is on his own and we have been told that we can do it up and put a flower container on it, but no headstone. This has been such a great comfort to me. I now know I really had a baby.'

Some parents, years after their baby's death, organise a ceremony to remember their baby, either alone or sometimes with other bereaved parents. A ceremony like this can help parents to begin to accept a loss which may have gone unmourned for many years. Helen and Stuart lost their second son, Luke, when Helen was twenty-one weeks pregnant. Luke was diagnosed as having Edwards' syndrome — a chromosomal abnormality — and they decided to terminate the pregnancy. Eight months after this, Helen miscarried another baby at eleven weeks. Even after the birth of a healthy daughter, Sarah, two years after Luke's death, Helen still felt unable to deal with her grief for Luke:

'Eventually I decided to go back to the hospital to ask all my unanswered questions. I cried non-stop for the two hours of my first meeting with the hospital counsellor, as she gently got me to relate all the pain I felt at never seeing Luke or having a photo. And not knowing how to remember him. She read out parts of the post-mortem which I had hardly heard at my six-week check and this cleared up some of the awful images I had of him. I found out that the baby I had miscarried was a girl. Finally, to my surprise, I found myself agreeing that I had always deep down wanted a service of remembrance.'

The hospital counsellor continued to help and support Helen and Stuart in the time up to the service, preparing them to let go and say goodbye to both their lost babies. The two of them were able to talk together about Luke as they had not done before, and Helen especially felt that she was no longer grieving alone. The service was conducted by the hospital chaplain:

'He began a simple service and as I heard the familiar prayers, the 23rd Psalm, my weeping subsided. He mentioned Luke and the little girl again and again and talked of their value despite their brief existence. Profound gratitude swept over me to know they were being acknowledged at last.'

This belated ceremony was a release for both Helen and Stuart. Two months later, Helen wrote that she could now look to a future 'where I will know how to remember the two babies lost with sadness but not with a burden of grief'. For some parents, such a ceremony can provide comfort and relief even ten or twenty years after the death of their baby.

## EXPRESSING GRIEF

To hold a funeral, or to go through some kind of ritual, public or private, is a way of expressing grief. But this is just one occasion, and there is a need, day by day and week by week, to continue to express feelings about the baby and to remember. To do this, it helps to have some focus for grief.

Parents who have a grave to visit know that they can, if they wish, go there and remember their baby whenever they need to do so. Others who do not have a grave or memorial to go to have a special place which they connect with their baby's memory — a favourite place or corner where they feel they are 'permitted' to give time to their baby's memory and to their own feelings. Some parents plant a tree or a rose bush in their garden, or keep fresh flowers in a special vase. Some have a particular place which they are fond of, where they can sit or walk and 'be with' their baby.

Mementos of their baby are very important to bereaved parents and can help them to focus their grief. They value anything and everything which can help them remember their child — a lock of hair, photos, a name tag, a cot card, foot and hand prints, stills from a scan. Judy spent time making an album in remembrance of her twins, using all these mementos:

> 'The album is very beautiful and special and is something we will treasure for the rest of our lives. It contains twelve photos of our twins in the special care baby unit, their birth and baptism certificates, congratulation cards, sympathy cards that we received after their death, all their birth details such as time, weight, length, etc., some poems and drawings, and a photo of their grave. It gave me great comfort making it and it gives us a permanent reminder of our babies' short lives. When we look through it together, it makes us feel very lucky that we were parents of our beautiful babies, even if it was for such a short time.'

Parents who do not have these mementos to treasure may find it hard to grieve, but sometimes it is possible to create some kind of personal remembrance book, containing, for example, photos taken during the pregnancy, cards people sent, favourite poems or other pieces of writing, an account of all that happened during the pregnancy and afterwards, some pressed flowers, and so on.

Creating a way of remembering a baby can itself be comforting because it means concentrating on the baby and giving him or her time.

Mementos can also be helpful in getting others to recognise and talk about the baby. Judy sent copies of her twins' photos to her family and this enabled everyone to acknowledge their deaths:

> 'Both our families coped with our tragedy by never mentioning it. We found this confusing and frustrating as it made us feel that it was all in our minds and we shouldn't be dwelling on it. But a couple of weeks ago I had a few reprints of our twins' photos done and we gave them to our parents, sisters and brothers and their families. It enabled us to open the subject with them, and we talked about the twins. Once everyone saw that we could talk about them calmly and without getting upset, they now mention them often.'

At some stage in their grieving, most parents need to talk, however difficult it is to do so. They need to talk about what happened, about their baby, and about their grief. At first, this need can be very strong. During the first weeks and months, some parents want to talk about their baby constantly. But it can be difficult to find listeners:

> 'My family and friends were all supportive in one way or another but nearly all found it very difficult to talk about it to me. I wouldn't broach the subject because I would just start to cry when I did. I knew it was an embarrassment to people, that they didn't want to upset me. A woman I knew through the National Childbirth Trust, whose baby had died the year before, came to see me as soon as she heard, a plant in one hand, a mass card in the other, no kids and free for the morning. She sat and talked with us for about two hours: it was wonderful.'

For many there is a need to go on talking, at least from time to time, over many years. As time passes, it can become even more important to remember and acknowledge the baby whom others have forgotten, or at least no longer mention:

> 'Even nine years on, I find I still need to talk to friends about Martin every now and then. In fact, the more years that go by, the more I feel I need to remember him. I am still in touch with one woman I met in hospital when Martin died. Her baby survived, but she's the friend I need because she's part of Martin's story and understands about him.'

Sometimes parents hold back from expressing their grief because they feel that others will think them morbid for continuing to think so much about their baby, or because they discover that people are embarrassed and cannot respond. Outsiders may particularly discourage tears — although a lot of parents know that it can be a great relief to cry. A month after her son Charlie's death, Kim found herself dwelling constantly on him and frequently in tears. Her photos of her son were a prompt, helping her to cry when she needed to, but she needed reassurance that to cry in this way was permissible and right:

> 'My GP said it would help me to put the photos out and not lock them away. This I've done. I've put the photos in frames on my walls and I feel really proud of them, but at the same time I feel very upset and I'm often in tears every time I look at them. My family tell me to take them down, but if I did this I would feel so guilty shutting my baby away. And I must admit, I feel so much better after a cry.'

Sometimes parents find other ways of expressing their grief — often by writing. Some write about their pregnancy and their baby's birth and death, some write poems or keep a diary. Many of the parents who have contributed to this book have said that it helped them to write about what happened and to think about their baby and their feelings, both then and now.

## GRIEVING TOGETHER, GRIEVING APART

Some couples feel very isolated in their grief and this sense of isolation from the rest of the world draws them closer together. They understand each other's grief in a way that no outsider can, and their shared memories of their baby are a strong tie. Peter and Christa depended on each other in this way in the time immediately after the death of their twin daughters. Peter writes:

> 'Losing the twins so suddenly, unexpectedly and traumatically was a very painful and profound shock. We had to be nursed and nurse ourselves together very gradually through the first few weeks. The normal world seemed far away and the first few short trips out of the

house were unpleasant. We clung to each other emotionally and talked about it a lot.'

Connie and Alan could also talk, and talking together helped them through:

'Alan and I have always been able to talk and that means an awful lot when you can talk to each other. We've been very fortunate in that way in that whatever happened we could talk about it.'

Connie and Alan lost four babies, twins first of all, and then later, two sons who were both born very prematurely. Connie's pregnancies were therefore increasingly stressful, and she depended very much on Alan's understanding:

'I know when Simon was on the way and I was starting to lose the baby, I was really angry and I expressed myself in a way that Alan could hardly believe. I screamed and I yelled, "Why is it happening again?" "What am I doing wrong?" "Why can't I hold on to my babies?", and he just sat and let me yell it all out, he understood.

'I was told I'd have to lie down for the whole of the pregnancy, and my first reaction was "I'm not lying down". And he understood, he wasn't angry. It's a tremendous help and a tremendous support, and I hope I've been the same to him. If he wanted to cry, I was there, and when I wanted to cry, he was there.'

But even in the closest relationships, it is sometimes hard for couples to comfort and support each other. Both partners are grieving, both are caught up in their own thoughts and feelings, and neither may be able to find the strength to attend to the other's needs or even be fully aware of how he or she is feeling. Often a couple's needs conflict, so that on a day when one partner feels particularly low, the other may be feeling less so. Patterns of grief often differ like this and as a result each partner can feel that they are struggling with their grief alone.

Sexual relationships can also be problematic. For some parents, making love is a comfort, but others cannot think of having intercourse for a long time after their baby's death. Quite apart from the difficulties which women normally experience after any birth (soreness, discomfort and uncertainty), after a baby's death there can be other feelings which are hard to deal with. Rosalind both did, and did not, want to make love:

'I desperately wanted to make love as soon as possible to cancel out the feeling that my body was some kind of coffin because she had died there, but I also felt I never wanted to again because she was the last person to be inside me and I didn't want to wipe out any part of that sacred memory. I was, and am, glad that my relationship with Tom was an old and firm one that could withstand the difficulties.'

Pat found that making love revived memories of her twins' birth and death. She was able to talk to her husband about how she felt but realised he felt differently:

'Every time we make love I relive the birth of the twins. I see Rebecca's brown, tiny body being resuscitated next to me, I hear both their cries as they were born — I relive it all. Usually I end up silently crying, but hide this from my husband. I'm better than I was in the few weeks after I came out of hospital and I have talked to my husband about everything I am feeling, even about my reaction to him in bed, and he understands enough for it not to be putting a strain on our love for each other, but I don't think he feels the same.'

For many couples, talking things through is very hard. Many are distressed to find that at the very time when they need each other most, they cannot be close to each other, and some find that their grief actually pulls them apart. Mary and Richard found that they dealt with their grief in very different ways. Their son, George, lived for five days:

'We grieved very differently. He tried not to think about it and hated talking about it. I was obsessed with talking about it. I would thrust George's photo at people and damn their embarrassment. I'm amazed we stayed together during the year after George's death. We could easily have been divorced.'

Hayriye and Şenol also went through a difficult time. Their son, Serdar, lived for twelve weeks. He was very ill and never left hospital. During that time, Hayriye and Şenol had frequent rows, and Hayriye felt bitter because she thought it was a time when they should have been close. After Serdar's death, Hayriye needed to cry and talk, but Şenol did not want to express his feelings openly and was unable to talk with her. Hayriye found this hard, and it led her to misinterpret Şenol's feelings about the death of his son:

'After Serdar died, I saw Şenol cry about twice. He wouldn't talk to me even though I needed to talk desperately. He seemed to be over it, while I was down and depressed. This went on for a long time. When I cried, he'd come to comfort me and I'd push him away. We were very distant, I think because we didn't talk and understand one another. I honestly thought we would separate. I used to talk about divorce a lot. Şenol said I was making life unhappy, I was spoiling our life. I said he'd better leave then. All the time he was being practical, working, bringing in the money, paying the bills, keeping us from going under that way. But all this was extremely petty to me.'

Şenol felt he should be strong and supportive, but this looked to Hayriye like insensitivity. Over a year later, Şenol described his feelings at the time of Serdar's illness and death:

'When Serdar was born and we were told of his brain damage, I felt in a totally different world, lonely, depressed and shocked. I had to be brave and support my wife, but as weeks went by I sank even lower. It was affecting me at work and at home. Friends at work were supportive; I was given compassionate leave for a while. They even had a collection for us so that I could take my wife out for a meal, and sent flowers too. When I did return to work (I'm a mechanic), I was given light duties for a time. I was at work physically, but mentally in deep thought about Serdar, my wife, our future.

'My inside felt shattered, crying internally so as not to show my emotions outside. I felt alone, without any support for me while I had to carry on to support my wife and hide my emotions.'

Hayriye was helped by finding others to whom she could talk, and in time this also eased the strain on her relationship with Şenol. After Serdar died, Hayriye's health visitor visited her for an hour each week to give her a chance to talk:

'That time was for me to pour out my grief to someone who didn't object to my tears or tell me what I should or should not do.'

Hayriye also met other bereaved parents in a local group. There, she was able to talk and be listened to, and she heard about other people's experiences. The meetings provided her with the kind of support she had looked for from Şenol but which he could not give, and also enabled her to understand his different way of grieving:

'The meetings have helped me a lot because these people have been in your shoes, they know what you are saying. My husband refused to come along, so I'd go alone. I came to understand that we were grieving in opposite ways. His was an inward, silent grief and mine was outward and apparent. The silence didn't mean he didn't care, it was just his way of grieving. He did get angry a few times when I kept on at him about not caring and forgetting. He told me he felt very angry inside.'

The expectations which society has of men can make it difficult, even unacceptable, for them to express their grief openly. Many grieve privately and more or less in silence. They may feel that their role is to keep normality going as far as possible, to take the practical strain, and to protect their partners. Many women, on the other hand, feel a pressing need to talk over events and discuss their feelings, and many are frustrated or perplexed by their partner's restraint. As a result, there can be misunderstandings on both sides, anger and arguments, with neither partner really understanding how the other needs to grieve or how best to give comfort or support.

It is not inevitable that men and women should grieve differently, but it is understandable if they do. There is much that a mother and father share when their baby dies, but their physical experience of loss is different: they lose different expectations, a different future, a different image of themselves. They are, in any case, separate individuals who will feel and express their emotions, including grief, in individual ways. When a relationship is put under stress after a baby's death, different ways of grieving, or different patterns of grief, can sometimes push it to breaking point. Many couples face the possibility of separation, and for some it becomes a reality.

Laura and Thomas's daughter, Katie, died; her twin sister, Hannah, survived. From the twenty-fourth week of pregnancy, Laura and Thomas knew that one of their twins would certainly die, but nobody could tell them when. It was hoped that the other twin would live. There were many weeks of stress and uncertainty which, along with their grief for Katie, eventually told on their relationship:

'We felt we had lost each other along the way, in fact we talked about separating. Our energies were low, and we weren't sure if we had it in us to work through the whole awful mess. I had such feelings of guilt and failure, I was angry and felt I had lost control of my life. Thomas was faced with an impotence he had never before experienced. He felt helpless and he too felt he had failed.'

In this situation, when both partners feel overwhelmed by their grief, and for that reason quite unable to reach out to each other, it can be important to get outside help. Laura and Thomas looked for the counselling they felt they needed:

'We decided to see a counsellor. We went once a week for six months and I'm glad to say we are happier together now and more in tune with each other than we have been for years. The counselling gave us both permission to express all kinds of feelings that were uncomfortable for us. That wasn't easy, in fact it was painful and it meant giving a lot of ourselves. But for us it was a positive step.'

Counselling is not a magic solution and it cannot eliminate differences. But a trained counsellor can provide one or both partners, either separately or together, with the chance to talk about and understand their own and each other's feelings. It may then become possible to find ways of dealing with difficulties which could otherwise cause a relationship to collapse. In some areas, counselling is offered to all parents whose baby dies; more commonly, parents themselves have to find the courage to recognise the importance and legitimacy of their needs — and the confidence to ask for what they think will help them. More information about counselling and how to obtain it can be found on pages 106–7.

## BROTHERS AND SISTERS

Children are often deeply affected by the death of a baby brother or sister and they too may need to grieve. But it can be hard for parents, in the midst of their own grief, to know how best to help.

Each child reacts differently to a baby's death and their needs vary. Parents too have different ways of responding to their children and what is an appropriate way for one family to cope is not necessarily right for another. But some understanding of other families' experiences can be helpful.

Even very young children are aware when their parents are upset, even when attempts are made to conceal distress, so they share in their parents' grief at least a little and have a need to understand something about the cause. Penny L's son, Adam, was 2 years old when his brother, Nicholas, died. Nicholas was born prematurely and lived in hospital for five and a half months. Adam was able to visit his brother and knew a lot about him by the time he died. When the hospital phoned at 6 o'clock one morning to say that Nicholas was deteriorating, Penny and her husband took Adam with them to the hospital. Nicholas was dead when they arrived:

'That day I didn't tell Adam that Nicholas had died. He was with us when we held Nicholas and he asked why we were crying, but I couldn't bring myself to tell him. For the week after that, my main worry was what we were going to say to Adam when he asked about Nicholas — but he didn't ask. Eventually the GP said we should raise the subject ourselves, so I screwed up my courage and told Adam that Nicholas had died and wasn't with us any more. From then on, Adam started asking a lot of questions.

'I now leave Nicholas's things around deliberately, so that we can talk. Adam doesn't get upset. He asks questions in a low-key way, so I don't get upset answering them. He often asks, "Where is Nicholas?" At first I didn't know how to answer this, but eventually I said he'd gone to heaven. I couldn't say that he was in the earth, or anything like that. That's hard enough for me to think about, let alone him. My GP and health visitor told me that Adam would have forgotten about Nicholas's death in a couple of months. But he doesn't forget, and I wouldn't want him to anyway.

'It was a great help to me that I came across two other women who had children about the same age as Adam and they had also had babies who died. We supported each other, and it helped me to be able to talk to Adam about those other deaths, so that he knew it was not only his baby who had died.'

Finding ways of talking about the baby who has died and answering children's (often very difficult) questions demands a great deal of courage and patience. It is a hard task for parents who are already emotionally exhausted. Many also fear breaking down in front of their children and feel that this will upset them more. But for most children unexplained silences and unanswered questions are much more difficult to accept than tears. Pat's son,

William, was 4 years old when his twin sisters were born prematurely and died. William was very upset, and Pat and her husband, Bob, had difficulty in finding satisfactory answers to his questions:

> 'He saw the girls in hospital, all tubed up, and we told him they were poorly. He wanted to know about the tubes and we told him they had tummy ache. This proved a bad thing later when he got tummy ache and thought he was going to die. He was at the hospital when Rebecca died but the nurses looked after him whilst Bob and I said goodbye to her. We told him they had gone to sleep and Jesus had taken them. This made him worry about sleeping for a time. He kept insisting he had not seen Jesus at the hospital so how could he look after them if he was not there.
>
> 'The worst time was two days after I came home. He turned to me and said if I was home where were his sisters, why had I left them behind? I explained they had died and he burst into tears and pushed me away from him.
>
> 'He has seen the grave and spent ages playing doctors and nurses and being dead. Offputting to other mums who have heard him, but obviously a comfort to him as now, eleven weeks after the twins' death, he seems to have accepted it very well.'

Small children who cannot put their feelings into words may express grief, and maybe bewilderment and anxiety, in the way they behave. This can result in difficult behaviour, just when parents feel least able to cope with it. Children also often use play to express themselves and to reach some understanding of events. Playing at doctors and nurses, at being pregnant and having a baby die, and similar games can help them, though they may be upsetting or irritating for their parents.

Older children may also go through a time of difficult, even unacceptable behaviour, becoming moody or clinging, having tantrums, refusing to sleep or refusing to co-operate. Patricia B's daughter was 7 when Patricia's second premature baby died:

> 'Her bereavement has followed a similar pattern each time, her aggression and attention-seeking not reaching its peak until four months after the event. Both times it has become apparent through her taking small items from myself and from other children, such as rubbers, money, small toys, a watch and a school recorder. This timing coincided with an improvement in my own physical and mental health so that I was less dependent on her for my own comfort (I needed

her to compensate for my loss), and my gradual regaining of self-confidence and independence so that I had less time to give her my attention. Each time it has taken us both a year to settle into a harmonious pattern of life.'

Children who are old enough to understand, more or less, what has happened will certainly feel their loss and also their parents' loss, and they may feel it acutely. Like their parents, they may have many complicated feelings to cope with, and at first they may find the death of their brother or sister impossible to accept. Like their parents they may need to go through a lengthy period of grieving, expressing how they feel and finding ways in which they can accept and come to terms with their loss.

Patricia A's children, David, aged 7½, and Julie, aged 6, were told by their father that their baby brother had been stillborn. They were both very upset and cried. The situation was made more difficult for them to cope with because they were unable to see their mother for some days after Paul Matthew's death. They thought that she was going to die too, and continued to worry about her for some time afterwards:

'Those first few weeks were the hardest. They needed so much love and attention. They were both tired, very demanding and had to be treated exactly alike. We also felt so protective of them and didn't want to tell them off when they needed it. We realised, though, they needed their normal routine back. We found that when it was "just the four of us" again, they settled down more.

'I suppose in a sense we are now over the worst as those weeks are behind us. But I feel angry when people say children soon forget. They may "bounce back" faster than we will, but the sadness, grief and multitude of other emotions are still there and will be there for many years to come. We may not talk about Paul Matthew as often but we still talk about him and questions and comments still occur. Julie suddenly said last week that it was all God and Jesus's fault that our baby had died, and how do you answer that? She is still obviously trying to come to terms with it all. They both comment on every baby they see, and quite often they say "I wanted our baby" and "why did he have to die?" — questions that we've asked ourselves time and time again. How do you answer your children when you don't always know the answers? All we feel we can do is be as open as we can and always be there for them.'

Children appreciate honesty and can become confused if they are misled. But some questions (such as 'Why did our baby have to die?') are impossible to answer because parents are themselves searching for the answers. Some parents are able to explain their baby's death in religious terms, and this is often easily accepted by children, but others feel uncomfortable with these explanations or simply cannot use them. They then have to find their own language to reassure their children and answer their questions.

Rosalind's daughter, Anna, was 7 when her sister, Georgia, was stillborn. She had already experienced the fun and happiness of the birth of a younger brother, Charlie, and she was looking forward to the new baby's birth, hoping that it would be a girl. Her grief over Georgia's death was hard for Rosalind to cope with:

> 'It is easy to underestimate how much children feel. They heal quicker than adults, but their grief is as intense. When Georgia died, my daughter, Anna, suffered so much that I still find it hard to talk about without crying.
>
> 'A couple of weeks before the birth I'd been told that the baby was small for dates so I'd warned the children that I might have to stay with the baby if it was kept in hospital. Anna asked if it would die, like a baby we'd heard of nearby. "No, of course not," I said. I regretted that so much in the months to come. "You promised me," she cried. "You promised me the baby wouldn't die. I hate you." Her grief was extreme and took over our lives.'

Rosalind found she could not put her own grief aside in order to help Anna with hers, and although she did try, she ended up feeling that she could have done better. In fact, by sharing some of the responsibility with others, Rosalind did eventually find the help Anna needed:

> 'Her teacher at school was wonderful and read books on bereavement and really tried to take on what I couldn't manage, but we still had a very disturbed little girl. She was bullied at school, and refused to go to school eventually. We had meetings with mothers of the bullies, who couldn't see why she should have special treatment. In the end, my health visitor referred her to a psychologist, who somehow worked wonders in six visits. Also, Anna was moved into a different class.'

Often children need people outside the immediate family — maybe a grandparent, a close family friend who they know and trust, a teacher or other professional — to give them support and help them cope with what they feel and what they see their parents feeling. Most children cope well with shared, family grief, and most manage better if feelings are honestly expressed rather than hidden. All children need their parents' love, and the reassurance that that love continues. But many also need some respite from their parents' distress, and an alternative, dependable source of comfort and support — and normality.

Parents cannot grieve *for* their children, or take away their grief or upset. This can be hard for parents to accept and many feel very helpless and inadequate. They are likely to have been able to comfort their children about any loss or hurt in the past and it is distressing to find that they cannot do the same now. Often mothers and fathers feel that if only they can answer their children's questions in the 'right' way, or say and do the 'right' things, then their children will not suffer. Yet parents also know that there are no satisfactory answers to their own questions, no instant cure for their own grief — and that the same is true for their children.

## FINDING SUPPORT

Some people need to grieve privately and have little need of contact with others. But at some point in their grieving, most parents are helped by contact with another person or other people who can understand what has happened and how they feel, and who can offer some kind of support. Family and friends cannot always help. Many parents find that even those closest to them are unable to understand or listen. Sue M was shocked to find that some of her closest friends had no understanding of her feelings after the death of her daughter:

'After my six-week check-up, a close friend came to see me. I was feeling very low and really wanted to be alone or to talk only with someone who understood. She kept asking, "Do they say you can try again?" and when I said yes, she said "Oh, isn't that wonderful, now you can forget the past and try again." I can't begin to tell you the sheer frustration of her misunderstanding. This incident and a few others made me withdraw from people. I pushed the hurt as far down as I could and kept saying, "I'm OK."'

But Sue was aware that there were some friends who could help her and that she needed their support:

'I withdrew from the friends who could not cope and relied more on the ones who could — the ones I could talk to and get helpful reactions from and be totally honest with. I asked them to help me by listening to me and letting me cry when I wanted to, and just being there when I needed them. One friend, Heather, who has been a great help, has a 4-month-old baby. I kept thinking that Nicky was the last baby I held and really wanted contact with babies again. So I asked Heather if I could call on my own and hold her baby. I said I might cry and feel sad. So after playing with her baby and holding her, I just let the tears come. This was such a help.'

But even those parents who are supported by their family and friends often find that a time comes when they need other help. They feel that they cannot continue to share their grief with the people who are close to them over a long period of time, yet their need to talk and express their grief goes on. Many find it helpful to have contact with other parents who have been through similar experiences and who therefore have a special understanding to offer:

'I had a wonderful husband and family, but you need to talk to others who have suffered in the same way, to know that the feelings you are experiencing are normal, and that you are not some kind of freak.'

Usually parents know when they need support. But it can be hard to summon up the courage and determination to make contact and ask for what is needed. It usually helps to have information about the kind of support available, and to know what other parents have done in similar situations.

Parents can make contact with local groups of bereaved parents through many of the organisations listed on pages 245–51, at any point in their bereavement. Some organisations offer group support, some also offer one-to-one befriending and telephone support. Parents can phone or write to find out what is available in their area. They can make contact, and maybe attend one or two meetings, without any commitment, to find out whether what is offered is right for them.

Alice did not feel in need of any outside support for some time after her daughter, Sarah, died. But as the first anniversary of Sarah's death approached, and at the beginning of another pregnancy, Alice began to find it hard to cope and decided to get in touch with her local group of the Stillbirth and Neonatal Death Society (SANDS):

> 'I wondered whether they would think me silly to phone almost a year after Sarah's death. But having plucked up the courage to go to a group meeting, I found I wasn't unusual. There were parents there whose babies had died many years before. What I got from that meeting was what I most needed, though I hadn't realised how much I needed it. I felt that my loss was accepted. I felt reassured that what I was feeling was normal, and that I could and would survive it. I felt I could talk (though it was hard at first), and that what I said was understood.'

Much later, as their own needs diminish, parents may want to help run a group or become a befriender themselves. For many this is an important way of making sense of their experience. Rosalind knew that she would not be able to help others until she had found a degree of equilibrium in herself, but in the meantime, her contact with SANDS gave her real hope:

> 'I wanted to share some of the self-knowledge I'd gained so tortuously by helping other people who had lost a baby, but I couldn't do it straight away. I was too raw and I would have bled with them. I'm still not very good at it: everyone's story makes me cry inside. But it's worth doing because I remember what a lifeline it was for me to see Rebecca who came to visit me after Georgia died, and to hear about her children who died. "How can you look so normal?" I asked her. She burst out laughing and I realised that maybe I wouldn't spend the rest of my life in a dressing gown with swollen eyes and uncombed hair.'

Some parents feel that they need professional support and sometimes it is easier to ask for what is needed from people whose job it is to provide it. Talking to an outsider can feel less stressful and help parents to look at things more calmly, from a distance.

Professionals such as GPs, community midwives and health visitors are now more aware of parents' need for support. In some areas, regular home visits are made in the time after a baby's death, usually by the community midwife or health visitor, to give parents the chance to talk about their baby's death and their own feelings, and to ask questions. Alternatively, parents can contact these professionals and explain the kind of help that they are looking for themselves. The quality of support that is offered will vary according to the individual professional concerned. Some are more experienced, more understanding, and able and willing to offer parents more time than others. However, at the very least, the GP, community midwife or health visitor should be able to supply information about local support groups, and about local bereavement counselling services.

Counselling means talking in confidence to an understanding outsider who is trained to listen and to help. It gives parents the opportunity to concentrate on their own feelings, to see and understand them more clearly, and to find their own ways of dealing with their grief. Knowing that the listener is both professional and an outsider can make it possible to air problems which may otherwise be difficult to talk about.

Some parents become aware many months or years after their baby's death that they need this kind of professional help. Some feel trapped by their grief, unable to deal with it alone and unable to move on. Others face particular difficulties — perhaps in their relationship with their partner or other children, or in adapting to a loss which has been particularly traumatic.

Peta was not offered counselling after her daughter, Emily, was stillborn. Looking back on her experience later, she knew that counselling would have helped her, but at the time she did not feel capable of seeking it herself. For three years she continued to feel bitter and upset, and never seemed able to grieve fully. But after the birth of her son, Oliver, she finally had the counselling she felt she needed:

'At last, after having counselling, I can honestly say the process is coming to an end and I feel "lighter". I hope I will now be able to place Emily as a beautiful memory, instead of the painful bitter thoughts I have surrounding her birth. It will always be sad, and leave a hole in the corner of my life. I can never say I am a 100 per cent happy. But it has taken only two months to stop the hurt I've had for three years.'

There are hospitals that now routinely offer counselling of some kind to all parents whose baby has died, perhaps through a hospital chaplain, midwife or social worker, or through a trained bereavement counsellor. Counselling may be offered at regular intervals over a period of time after the baby's death, or it may be available as and when it is felt to be needed. Services like this are patchy, but increasing.

Those who feel that they would benefit from counselling should also be able to obtain information about counselling services in their area through their GP. Some GP practices have counsellors attached to the practice. Other GPs will refer parents for counselling, perhaps with a professional counsellor, or through a local bereavement service manned by trained volunteers. In a few areas, where services are good, parents can make direct contact with a counselling service themselves. Local libraries and Citizens Advice Bureaux can usually provide information about these local services, and the British Association for Counselling (address on page 248) can give information about counselling services around the country. Some but not all of these services are free.

## 'WILL I EVER GET OVER IT?'

'Somebody said to me it's something you get over, but I've never felt that. I've always felt that if you're lucky, you come through. There are times when you're going through it when you think it will never end, you'll never ever come through it, you'll never enjoy anything again and you can't go on. Then one day the bad days and the despair begin to lift and gradually you know that you are going to make it. I can remember smiling again and thinking, "I'm smiling!" And having been sure I'd never smile again.'

Parents do not 'get over' their baby's death. Most do not expect to, nor do they want to forget their baby or any of the events connected with their baby's life and death. All know that they will carry some sadness with them for the rest of their lives. But they also hope that they will eventually come to terms with their loss, find some way of living with it, and find it possible to be happy again.

For most parents, this hope is realised. In time, they become able to accept what has happened, and to think about their baby calmly, with a much quieter sadness, as well as with love. There may still be bad times, but the bad times become fewer, and the times between become better. Three and a half years after her twin daughters died, Christa felt that her sadness was still there but had changed:

> 'I can now say that by and large I have come to terms with the loss of my daughters. The sadness I feel now is a tribute to them. I still do get those awful bad days when the pain is as great as it was in the beginning, but thankfully these days are few and far between. I never thought in the early days that we could find happiness again, but we have.'

But it is not only the passage of time which enables parents to adapt to their loss. There is also a need to work at grief, a need to grieve actively, a need to mourn. Grief which is stifled or hidden or ignored, in whatever way and for whatever reason, does not ease.

It takes some parents more time, some less to go through the process of mourning their loss. There is no prescribed time-scale, just as there is no set pattern to grief. But almost all parents find that grieving is harder, and takes longer, than they ever expected; and that it is sometimes harder, and takes longer, than they think they are able to bear. Many reach a stage when they feel that they should be feeling better, but are not. They feel exhausted by their grief, forgotten by their friends who no longer acknowledge their loss, and convinced that their sadness will never lessen. Some think that they must be abnormal to continue to grieve for what seems to be such a long time; they feel as though they are ill without hope of recovery.

Angela's daughter, Suzanne, died twenty-eight hours after birth: her story is told on page 11. Almost a year and a half later, Angela lost her next baby when she was eight weeks pregnant. After this second loss, Angela felt that she could no longer cope.

But this miscarriage proved a turning point. For a time Angela was in despair, but then she came to understand that her grief was unavoidable and that grieving was a necessary task, no matter how daunting it is:

> 'I was wanting and hoping for a way out of my grief, but now I realise there's no way out of it or around it. I've got to go through it whether I like it or not. I also realise that I still have a long way to go, perhaps three steps forward and one step back sometimes.'

A month after this, Angela wrote:

> 'The pain is indescribable. You have to have been there to know just how it feels. If we look back, we've been through hell, and we've done well to survive. But we can do it and have done it so far. It gives me a strange sense of achievement that I'm not going to ruin my life or my family's, that we are going to get through this, despite the pain and the agony.'

# 5  Another Pregnancy

Most bereaved parents, either straight away or after a time, face a decision about whether and when they will have another baby. They also face all the questions, anxieties and real risks that this decision can bring. This chapter looks at parents' feelings before and during another pregnancy, and also at antenatal care in a pregnancy that follows the loss of a baby.

For a very few parents, there is no possibility of another pregnancy. In some cases, medical problems make it impossible or too dangerous for the mother. In others, medical or genetic problems mean that the risk of another loss is too high for parents to contemplate. Even if there is no specific risk, some parents simply know that they cannot survive the stresses and worries of another pregnancy that might again end in disaster.

Although this happens to very few parents, for those few the final realisation that there will be no more children can be very painful, and is often a new bereavement in its own right. Imogen had a stillborn baby at thirty-eight weeks and then had two miscarriages. She felt that in her case the chance of ever bringing a pregnancy to a successful conclusion was very slight, and that it would be better to make the decision to stop trying herself, rather than to expose herself to the likelihood of further loss and devastating pain. But for her this decision brought a double grief: she had not only lost her babies but also had to cope with losing the possibility of parenthood:

> 'I am 44 years old and I feel that as far as having babies is concerned time is running out for me. I felt it would be less painful if I took the decision into my own hands.'

Fiona S and her husband, Ron, lost four babies. With the prospect of intensive medical intervention in another pregnancy and no guarantee of a successful outcome, they too made the decision not to try again. Although this was very hard, in some ways it freed them to begin to move on and think about what they would make of their lives without children:

> 'We'd virtually spent ten years of our lives trying to have babies. Looking back, that was grim. I was watching my periods every month, we lost spontaneity, our love-life suffered — everything suffered because we were so preoccupied. It put a tremendous strain on us. And it did us both an enormous amount of good to finally make the decision not to go on. Coming to that decision was hard, but having made it was in some ways better.'

Parents who have lost one or more babies and are then childless are not always given recognition or sensitive support. Their situation is particularly hard and can be made worse because of other people's assumptions that either they have chosen not to have children or have never had any. Parents in this position can feel very isolated. Some may find it helpful to contact other parents who are childless. The National Association for the Childless and CHILD both offer support and contact with other parents who cannot have children and/or who have medical or fertility problems. People who are considering adoption or fostering may like to contact the British Agencies for Adoption and Fostering. See pages 249—50 for the addresses of all these groups.

## THINKING ABOUT ANOTHER BABY

Many bereaved parents feel an overwhelming urge to have another baby. Although they know that they cannot replace the baby who has died, and do not want to, they also long desperately for a living baby to love and to hold. They hope that another baby will help to fill the terrible emptiness they feel.

Barbara's baby was born prematurely at twenty-six weeks gestation and lived for only one day. Barbara had waited some time to start a family and had been very unsure whether she wanted a baby at all:

> 'I've spent my life not wanting children, or at least not being sure that I wanted them, and now, since my baby died, it's the only thing I

want — the only thing that'll make me happy. I can't think or really care about anything else.'

Diana already had a daughter, Lydia, when she gave birth to twins, Robert and Bryony. Robert was stillborn; Bryony was small but healthy. Having planned and made space in her heart for two new babies, Diana found herself longing to get pregnant again and to fill the empty space left by Robert's death:

> 'I knew, within a day of having our twins, that I wanted another baby. We'd always planned on just two children, but then when we were expecting the twins, our expectations, hopes and love were built up for three children, and now there was this aching void. The desire to have another baby was compounded by guilt and a lack of trust in my own feelings. When I voiced my longing I was met by disbelief and almost horror from family, especially my parents — surely I couldn't put myself through another trauma? So I kept quiet and hugged these feelings to myself.'

For parents whose confidence and self-esteem have been battered by their loss, having another baby may also be important for their own survival. At this time of intense grief and pain, it may be the one thing that they feel can restore their confidence in themselves and their sense of purpose and meaning in life. Surinder had two pregnancies that ended prematurely. Her whole life then became focused upon having another baby:

> 'After my second baby died it became nearly an obsession. I had to have another child. I knew that was what I needed more than anything.'

Sometimes parents worry that their urgent need to have another baby seems to conflict with their equally strongly felt need to treasure and honour the memory of the baby who died. They may fear that wanting to become pregnant again seems to deny the strength of their love for the baby who died, that they are looking onwards to the future when they should be holding on to the past.

For Jane, the idea of having another baby seemed out of the question for a long time. In Jemma she had lost the one baby she ever wanted. So when, ten months after Jemma was stillborn, Jane decided to try to get pregnant again, she worried that she was being somehow disloyal:

'Would she know that I had "discarded" her and chosen to have another baby just because her pregnancy was a "failure"? Would she know, somehow, that I'd apparently closed the book on her, after only a few months, and after all we'd been to each other?'

The loss of a baby often clarifies parents' priorities and gives them a heightened awareness of the importance of having and being a family. Isabel, whose first son was born prematurely and died two days later, writes:

'Most of all, we have a new and passionate commitment to parenthood. We really want another baby, not in the casual way of couples who take their ability to bear children for granted, but in the heartbreaking knowledge of the true value of a child's life. However many children we eventually have, there will always be one more than the census reveals: our first, much-loved and deeply-mourned son — Benjamin.'

Sometimes the intense longing simply to have and hold another baby begins to recede after a while, and parents' feelings become more complicated. Peta, for example, wanted another baby very badly but worried about how she would feel towards a baby who was not the daughter she had lost:

'At first I wanted a baby immediately, but now I want to wait a while, but no longer than six months. I'm afraid everyone will say I should wait a year — we will see. I must stop being upset. At present I worry I won't love another baby. It won't be so perfect, especially if it's a boy. I suppose once I'm pregnant I'll grow to love it too.'

Many parents fear that they simply would not survive if another baby were to die: 'The pain would be too overwhelming, you would just fade away.' Bereaved parents know only too well that all pregnancies carry some risk to the baby, however small. Tina B, whose first baby, Chloe, was stillborn, writes:

'Even though we have been told to try again after Christmas, I dread becoming pregnant again. I know that at the end of the day no one can guarantee us a baby, and I know that it is a chance we will have to take.'

Often there is pressure from friends and relations to get pregnant again. The parents' grief at the loss of their baby is clearly so painful, and their need for their baby so great, that it seems to those who care about them that only another baby can begin to heal the wounds. Tracie's baby, Darrel, was stillborn at thirty-seven weeks:

> 'My mum thinks I should have another baby as it will help me to come to terms with it. My boyfriend wants to have another baby too, and so do I in some ways, but I'm just so scared of this happening again. I can hardly cope now without bursting into tears every five minutes, but if this should happen again I think I would just die.'

There can be other pressures too. Women who are approaching the end of their childbearing years often feel that time is running out and are fearful either that they will not be able to conceive again or are taking a risk in trying to do so. Parents who already have an older child may very much want to have another baby as soon as possible so that there will not be too great an age gap in the family. Many women fear that they will not be able to conceive again.

Women who took a long time or had difficulty in conceiving the baby who died may have particular reason to feel such fear. They may want to talk to their GP or consultant early on about the possibility of referral for investigation at a specialist fertility clinic. Professionals have different views on the length of time that should elapse before fertility treatment is attempted. But for parents who have lost a baby, the need to have another may be particularly urgent and should be regarded sympathetically.

Sometimes parents' shared experience of grief and longing for the baby who died moves naturally into a shared decision to try for another baby. But sometimes the very question of whether or not to try again puts a relationship under strain. One partner may urgently need and want a baby; the other may feel that they simply cannot go through the worry and pressure of another pregnancy. Dora's baby, Edward, died in the womb the day before he was born. She and her husband already had one son, who was 3 years old at the time of Edward's death:

> 'I long for a baby — we've been trying, but nothing. My husband doesn't understand me, I can't talk to him. He says I'm stupid because

I want a baby so much. I long for a baby, a brother or sister for my son. My stomach yearns for a baby. My husband says it shouldn't dominate my life and that there are more important things — him and my son.

'I love my husband and my son so much. I try for my son's sake to keep happy and not to be miserable. I don't want a baby to replace Edward — no one ever would. I just want a baby.'

The grief and stress which follow a baby's death often cause a relationship to go through a very bad time, and it may then be difficult for parents to feel sure about embarking on another pregnancy, especially one that is likely to be more than usually stressful and anxious. Gloria, whose twins died in the womb at twenty-six weeks, felt that since the twins' deaths she and her husband had drifted apart:

'I'd love to try again, whatever the risks, but I'm not sure how long we'll stay together, we don't seem to agree on anything or have anything in common any more. I don't think it would be fair to bring a baby into such an uncertain situation.'

Sometimes making love can itself be a problem. Many parents find that their grief causes them to withdraw physically from each other:

'I would like to have more children but am afraid to. My sex-life has suffered. Sex to me means pregnancy and that means pain and death.'

Tina N's first baby, Sarah, was stillborn. Although she wanted another baby, she was frightened that everything might go wrong again. Subconsciously she avoided sex at the times when she was most likely to conceive:

'I realised that I was purposely having headaches around the time I could get pregnant. Then I would spend two days crying when a period happened. It was the fear of failing again.'

Some bereaved parents find that the question of whether to try for another baby and fear about the outcome fill most of their waking hours. The constant awareness and pain of their loss, and the reality of babies and children all around them, means that they can rarely stop turning the decision and the questions over in their minds. Rosie describes herself as normally very placid, but eight months after her baby's death she found herself absorbed with the question of another pregnancy, and also very confused:

'My problem now is that my common sense tells me I need another baby. I find myself looking at other babies and wanting them. Doctors and midwives, friends and relatives, all seem to think that the best possible course is to try again. But I seem to have a mental block against pregnancy. The slightest mention of morning sickness or anything else associated with pregnancy makes me go hot and cold all over. Last month my period was late and I was panic-stricken in case I was pregnant, I had diarrhoea for two days because I felt so physically sick at the thought of the possibility of being pregnant.

'On good days, when I'm feeling strong, I tell myself that I'm being stupid and another baby will put things in perspective, but the rest of the time I cringe from the pregnancy — not from the idea of the baby but from the nine months and not knowing whether I'll be luckier this time.

'All the people I know who have lost babies all seem only too eager to have another, and many seem to do so within twelve months of losing the previous one. I am in utter confusion, swinging from longing for a baby to being physically sick at the thought of being pregnant.'

One strategy that can help certain parents to regain some control over the situation is to decide for the moment to make no decision, and to set a date some time in the future to talk and try to work out what to do:

'We decided it was taking over our whole lives, the question of trying again, but at the same time we couldn't make a decision we felt right about. So we agreed to try not to think about it again till after our holiday, and we managed it most of the time. That gave us some space to think and talk about other things.'

Some parents are helped by some form of professional counselling. The opportunity, for example, to talk openly and honestly without fear of being judged may release some of the pressure of unhappiness and grief that they hold inside themselves. It may help them to find their way through a very difficult time, enabling them to feel stronger and more confident. Counselling can also be helpful for those couples who find that the loss of their baby has badly affected their relationship. In many places, hospital doctors and GPs can refer people for counselling. Alternatively, for a list of counselling organisations, see pages 248–9.

## MEDICAL FACTS THAT MAY INFLUENCE THE DECISION

All bereaved parents feel anxious and fearful about the prospect of another pregnancy. For some, especially if there is no reason to believe that problems will recur, the decision about trying again can be made when they are ready and on the basis of their own feelings.

But for other parents, particularly those who need to consider specific medical risks, deciding whether or not to try again can be very difficult and may require detailed discussion with sympathetic, well-informed professionals. Parents in this situation may want to discuss the known medical facts, the likely risks that another pregnancy would involve, and what could be done to diagnose and possibly treat any problems that arose in another pregnancy. Such discussion can help them make an informed decision and so take some control of their situation.

The first step may be to go over what happened before. Parents need to be sure that they understand everything they can about what happened and why their baby died. Even after a long time, it may still be possible to contact the obstetrician under whose care the pregnancy took place and/or the neonatologist who looked after the baby in special care, and to ask for a discussion of everything that happened. Even if the consultant is no longer at the hospital, all medical notes are usually kept for at least ten years, and it should be possible to arrange a meeting with another doctor in the right department to discuss what can be learned from the notes.

Sometimes a discussion about the likely risks in another pregnancy does not always help very much in terms of clear medical facts. There are still many gaps in medical knowledge about pregnancy and the development of babies in the womb, and in many cases even a post-mortem or other investigation cannot explain why a baby was stillborn or born prematurely. If this is so, it may be difficult to learn very much that is helpful about specific risks in another pregnancy. But it can still be useful for parents to be as clear as possible in their minds about any facts that are known and their implications. They may also like to discuss in detail, with the professionals involved, how another pregnancy would be monitored and what special care and support they would receive, as well as any other fears and anxieties they have.

If the cause of their baby's death *is* known, parents need to find out whether it is likely to recur in another pregnancy. If it is, it is clearly important to find out what could be done both before and during the pregnancy, to try to avoid or minimise problems and to plan the best possible management of the pregnancy. Parents may wish to discuss these questions at a specialist pre-pregnancy clinic or to ask their GP to refer them to a consultant with special experience in this area. They may also want to get in touch with a support or self-help group for advice and contact with other people in the same situation (see pages 246–8 for list of addresses).

If there seems to have been a genetic factor in their baby's death, the hospital will usually offer parents counselling with a genetic specialist – a doctor who can assess and discuss genetic risk in pregnancy. Parents can also ask their GP to refer them to a genetic specialist.

Some parents, having reviewed the medical facts, decide not to try for another baby. For them the risk of further loss is simply too great. The decision to stop trying can be very hard, but it can also mean an end to a period in their lives when they were under the constant strain of wanting something very badly and knowing they might never have it. It can seem better to remove this strain and to concentrate on other parts of their lives.

## GENETIC COUNSELLING

Genes in the egg and sperm cells that form the fertilised egg carry the information which determines how a baby will develop. In some cases, a baby's abnormal development in the womb is caused by abnormal inherited genes. This can happen either because the genes were accidentally reorganised when the egg and/or the sperm cells were forming, or because one or both parents carries a gene for a particular condition or disease (see below). A genetic specialist can usually tell parents if the problem is genetic and can discuss the risk of the condition recurring in a future pregnancy.

It is sometimes difficult to calculate the specific risk that a genetic condition will recur. The calculations depend partly on how much is known about the condition; they also depend on identifying how the baby inherited the condition, and this cannot always be done. The counsellor may need to take a detailed family history of both partners. It is worth being prepared for the appointment by obtaining details about any family members who might be relevant, for example, grandparents, brothers and sisters and cousins, if this can be done without upsetting the family.

## Ways in which a baby can inherit a condition
(See also page 202.)
**Single gene inheritance** A baby inherits two of each gene, one from the father and one from the mother. Certain genes can carry traits for specific conditions or diseases. Some genetic traits are *dominant*, which means that a baby only has to inherit an affected gene from one parent to have the condition. Brittle bone disease and tuberous sclerosis, for example, are dominant traits. If either parent carries a dominant trait in his or her genes, there is a 1 in 2 chance in each pregnancy that the baby will be affected.

Most genetic traits for serious or fatal conditions are *recessive*. This means that a baby will only inherit the condition if *both* parents carry the trait for the condition and if *both* parents pass on the affected gene at conception. If both parents carry a recessive trait, there is a one in 4 chance in each pregnancy that the baby will be affected (see fig. 1 and caption on page 120). This 1 in 4 risk applies to each pregnancy and is not altered by the number of affected or unaffected babies the couple has already had. Conditions that are inherited through recessive traits include sickle cell disease (see page 199), thalassaemia (see page 218) and cystic fibrosis.

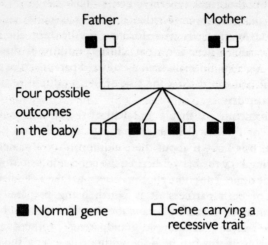

*Fig. 1* Diagram of recessive inheritance.

A baby inherits one gene from each parent. In *each* pregancy there is:

- a 1 in 4 chance that the baby will inherit two genes carrying the recessive trait and be affected
- a 1 in 4 chance that the baby will inherit two normal genes and be unaffected
- a 2 in 4 chance that the baby will inherit one gene carrying the recessive trait and one normal gene. The baby will be unaffected but may pass the condition on to his or her own children.

The chances in each pregnancy are not affected by the outcomes of earlier pregnancies.

Some conditions (known as X-linked conditions) are only carried by the woman but normally only affect male babies. Haemophilia, for example, is X-linked. If a woman carries an X-linked condition there is a one in 2 chance that each male baby will be affected. Female babies cannot normally be affected, but there is a one in 2 chance that each female baby will carry the gene for the condition and so could pass it on to her own children.

**Multifactorial disorders** Many conditions are caused by a combination of genetic and environmental factors. This means that one or both parents may carry a trait which carries a tendency for a particular condition. Whether a baby develops the condition also depends on certain external factors (most of which are not yet known) which may be present during the first few months in the womb. Conditions which are thought to arise as a result of a combination of genetic and environmental factors include neural tube defects (see page 205), some congenital heart abnormalities (see page 211) and Potter's syndrome (see page 216).

Where a condition is caused by a combination of genetic and environmental factors it is often more difficult for a genetic counsellor to assess the risk that it will recur. The risk is usually estimated on the basis of figures collected from other families with a similar problem.

**Chromosome abnormalities** Most developmental abnormalities are not caused by a specific gene that carries a hereditary trait or tendency down through the generations. Many arise when chromosomes accidentally become rearranged as the egg and/or sperm cell is formed. The baby then has abnormal chromosomes and develops abnormally. Conditions resulting from chromosome abnormalities include Edwards' syndrome, Patau's syndrome, and Down's syndrome (see pages 204–5).

This accidental rearrangement of chromosomes is most commonly a one-off accident and is known as *non-disjunction* (see also page 204). The risk of non-disjunction in a pregnancy may be somewhat higher if a couple has already had a baby affected by non-disjunction, and may increase further as the mother gets older, particularly once she is over 40.

In a very few cases, one or both parents inherits a tendency to produce a fairly high proportion of egg or sperm cells with abnormally arranged chromosomes. This is known as *balanced chromosomal translocation* or, in some cases, *inversion* (see also page 204). In this case the risk of the couple having another baby with the same condition is always increased, though it varies for different chromosome rearrangements.

Even when parents can be given a precise numerical risk, for example, a one in 20 chance that another baby will have the same condition, individual parents have different feelings about what that risk means to them. If there is a one in 20 chance of a condition recurring, there are 19 out of 20 chances that it will not recur. In other words, out of every 100 women who face a one in 20 risk and who then go through another pregnancy, it is likely that 5 will have a baby with this condition and 95 will not. For some parents this may be a risk they are prepared to take, for others it may be unacceptably high.

Lorraine, who has a daughter, Mary, aged 5, and has had two stillbirths since Mary's birth, felt that neither she nor her family could cope with the possibility of another loss:

> 'The doctor said that in our case there was a one in 20 chance of the next baby dying so we have decided not to try again. We know that neither of us could survive another death, and we don't want to put Mary through any more disruption and unhappiness. She goes through it with us and she's been really affected. We've all had enough pain and we want to put our energy into looking after Mary and each other now and getting ourselves together as a family.'

Someone else, given the same statistical possibility, might decide it is worth going ahead. Like most decisions to do with being a parent, there are no right answers, only the answer that seems best for each person at the time.

## WHEN TO TRY AGAIN

Parents who want to consider the possible medical and emotional issues surrounding the timing of another pregnancy may find it helpful to go back to their GP or hospital consultant, or to a counsellor, to ask questions and have a detailed discussion. Decisions are hard to make without information, and professional advice can be helpful provided the professional concerned understands parents' strong feelings and emotional needs.

On purely physical grounds, doctors usually advise parents who are keen to try to conceive again that they should wait until the mother has had two or three normal periods and is back into a normal cycle. However, many professionals feel that bereaved parents benefit emotionally if they wait for longer, at least six months and possibly a full year, before embarking on another pregnancy. Although there is little scientific evidence on this issue, it is often believed that those parents who have had more time to focus fully on the baby who has died, and who have had a fairly long gap before the conception of another baby, are likely to find another pregnancy and the development of their relationship with another baby less difficult. Although these parents still continue to grieve and to feel the acute loss of the baby who has died, it may be easier for them to see the new baby as a person in his or her own right, both before and after the birth.

Many parents themselves are also aware that if another pregnancy begins very soon, the new baby may be born around the first birthday or anniversary of the baby who died. This is a time when they are likely to be particularly sad and distracted and when it may be difficult to feel much for the new baby. It may be harder not to feel that the new baby is a replacement for the one who died, or not to wish that the new baby *was* the one who had died.

However, after a baby has died it can be hard to think coolly and objectively about the timing of another pregnancy. Many parents want very much to get pregnant again as soon as possible, and, for them, that strength of feeling outweighs all other considerations. Rosalind, for example, whose daughter, Georgia, was stillborn, did not wait:

> 'I needed a baby, I wanted a live baby, and although I was told, and could see, that I needed time to heal and to grieve, I couldn't wait.'

Kim's second child, Charlie, was born prematurely and died after thirteen days in special care. Kim and her husband longed to start another pregnancy as soon as possible and were upset and angered when they were advised to wait. They felt that only they could know what was right for them, and they were prepared to cope with the consequences of their decision. To them, the advice they were given was unwelcome and intrusive:

> 'How I see it is that another baby never could or would replace our son, Charlie. We do realise what we are doing and that there is no way a new baby could or would become a substitute for Charlie.
> 'My son, Charlie, was wanted and conceived out of love, and our

next child will also be wanted and conceived out of love and not out of convenience, so why are people making my husband and myself feel bad for wanting to try for another baby so soon after Charlie's death? So many people have offered advice concerning this but it's up to us what we decide to do and we feel in our hearts that it's right to try for another baby.'

For Hayriye, over a year after the death of her son, Serdar, the time for another baby had not yet come:

'One day we would like to have another baby. But at the moment thinking about another child makes me cry for the one I've lost. But it is clear in my mind that Serdar was Serdar, his love and memory are separate. Another child will be our third child and another door in my heart. We can never replace someone who has died, it would not be right and I would not want to. The family keep telling me to have another baby and to forget, and to give my love to my other son, Serhan, and to a new baby. But each child's love is individual, just like themselves. I couldn't love a new baby instead of Serdar, but as well as. There are no limits to how much we can love.'

In the end, the timing of another pregnancy is an intensely personal decision and parents must be guided by their own feelings. Only they can know and weigh up all the different factors that will influence their decision. Only they can know their own strengths, needs, wishes and circumstances, and when it feels right for them to begin to move on to what will be a new relationship with a new baby.

## PREPARATION AND CARE DURING ANOTHER PREGNANCY

The decision to try for another pregnancy can bring with it a good deal of stress. Besides the constant anxiety that everything may go wrong again, it can take some time to conceive. There may be a long period of ups and downs, hope and then disappointment, elation and depression.

When and if a new pregnancy begins, parents often find themselves surprised at how difficult it can be. The joy and hope of a new pregnancy are frequently overlaid by worry and by renewed grief for the baby who died. For some parents, the pressures of this new pregnancy can lead to difficulties in their relationship; for others, the struggle to get through this pregnancy and the hope of success strengthens them as a couple.

It can help parents to find ways to manage the inevitable stresses of this time and to do what they can to increase their confidence and their physical and emotional well-being. The knowledge that they are reasserting some control over their lives and helping to try to ensure a successful outcome next time can be very important. Each person needs to find ways that are right for them, but often relatively simple measures can be helpful in getting through difficult times to come. Such measures may include, for example, eating a healthier diet, getting more exercise and fresh air, identifying and reducing the unnecessary stress in their lives, and consciously choosing to spend time doing things they enjoy.

It can also help to find someone, a relative, a friend or a professional perhaps, who will support them by listening uncritically to their feelings and their worries:

> 'I had been going for counselling before I got pregnant for the fourth time, and through the early months of the pregnancy. It was wonderful to have someone really to talk to and while I don't think counselling made me any better, it at least released some of the pressure that was building up inside me.'

Although it is indeed difficult to prove that counselling and other relatively simple measures alter the physical course of a pregnancy, they certainly do no harm to the new baby, and can only help the parents. For parents whose confidence and self-esteem have been brought low, it can be very important to put themselves back consciously in the centre of the picture where they belong, and to begin to care for and value themselves again.

## MEDICAL ADVICE

Many parents wish to discuss with their doctors and midwives what they can do to try to ensure that their new baby is born alive and well. However, except where a clear and treatable medical cause was found for the previous death, the advice parents receive often seems frustratingly negative and non-specific. There is good reason for this: as yet, very little is understood about what affects the development of a baby in the womb and about what general measures can be safely taken to assist and safeguard this development. For example, there is no evidence that special dietary supplements, taken on top of a basically healthy diet during or before pregnancy, benefit either babies or mothers, though it is known that certain vitamins taken in excess can do harm. What is clear is that it can be dangerous to interfere unnecessarily with the complex, interlinked processes that normally ensure the birth of a healthy baby, and that past efforts to do so have sometimes caused damage and usually had no beneficial effect.

Nevertheless, the fact that doctors and other professionals cannot meet the wishes of many parents for specific advice about how to try to ensure a successful outcome to the pregnancy, should not prevent them from listening to parents' worries and talking over possible courses of action.*

## TENDER LOVING CARE

A pregnancy after a baby has died is often very hard. Many parents find themselves filled with anxiety, self-doubt, unhappiness and confusion. Anything that they can do to relieve some of this stress will help to make the pregnancy a happier time. It is even possible that relieving stress may sometimes affect the physical progress and outcome of the pregnancy. For example, the body under stress produces hormones which can affect the uterine muscle and may be the reason why women under great stress have an increased risk of premature labour. Relieving stress may cut down or prevent the release of these hormones.

A study in Norway looking at a sample of women who had a history of three or more consecutive miscarriages, found that

---

*For a discussion of the latest scientific evidence on the general management of pregnancy and childbirth, including pre-pregnancy care, see Murray Enkin, Marc J.N.C. Keirse and Iain Chalmers, *A Guide to Effective Care in Pregnancy and Childbirth* (Oxford University Press, Oxford, 1989).

among those women who had no specific abnormality, increased individual care and support from the professionals looking after them seemed to double the success rate in their next pregnancy. This study compared women who received a lot of personal contact and care from the hospital in their next pregnancy, including weekly medical examinations but little or no medical treatment, with other women who got ordinary antenatal care elsewhere. Of those women who received increased individual care and attention (but not increased medical treatment) from the hospital, over twice as many had successful outcomes to their pregnancy.

Although the study was not a scientifically-controlled trial, the results are important and thought-provoking. At the very least the study should give bereaved parents the confidence to ask for a high standard of care and individual attention from professionals during the next pregnancy. It may also encourage them to ask for emotional support from their family and friends during their next pregnancy, and consciously to seek out and spend time with those people whom they find supportive and caring.*

## SMOKING

There is clear evidence that if a woman smokes during pregnancy her baby is likely to be affected. Smoking constricts the blood vessels and cuts down the blood supply to the placenta. The chemicals and gases in cigarettes can also prevent the baby growing properly. In addition, smoking can increase the risk of miscarriage, premature labour (see page 225) and placental bleeding and abruption (see page 182). By itself, smoking increases the risk to a baby only very slightly, but when it is

*B. Stray-Pedersen and S. Stray-Pedersen, 'Recurrent abortion: the role of psychotherapy' in R.W.Beard and F. Sharp (Eds), *Early Pregnancy Loss: Mechanisms and Treatment* (London: RCOG, 1988); also, B. Stray-Pedersen and S. Stray-Pedersen, 'Etiologic factors and subsequent reproductive performance in 195 couples with a prior history of habitual abortion' in *American Journal of Obstetrics and Gynaecology*, vol. 148, no. 2, January 1984.

combined with other factors that can also increase risk, such as a poor diet or poverty, and in some cases a previous stillbirth, miscarriage or neonatal death, it can dramatically increase the risk to the baby. Smoking by either partner may also make it more difficult for a couple to conceive.

Giving up smoking is hard: smokers who are addicted find it particularly difficult. People may also want and need to smoke when they are stressed and sad. Clearly it is best for both parents to stop smoking altogether if they can, preferably before a new baby is conceived. This will ensure that the baby develops in a cigarette-free environment. But for those parents who find it impossible to stop smoking, even just for the duration of their next pregnancy, research has shown that stopping or cutting down as much as possible *at any time* during the pregnancy will benefit the baby to some extent.

Parents who want to give up smoking before or during a pregnancy often find it easier if they can get outside help, for example, from their GP or a local stop-smoking group. For more information about ways of giving up smoking, contact QUIT (see page 250 for the address).

## ALCOHOL

The evidence to show that alcohol causes damage to a developing baby is far less clear than it is for smoking except in those cases where a woman drinks significantly more than 1oz of absolute alcohol a day. (1oz is, for example, four measures of spirits or four glasses of wine or two pints of beer or cider.) People who drink this much alcohol regularly are more likely to have a miscarriage. Their babies are also more likely to have major abnormalities, learning difficulties and to be small at delivery. (This combination of symptoms is known as fetal alcohol syndrome.) The effects of alcohol on a baby seem to be increased if the mother also smokes. Heavy drinking by either partner may also make it more difficult for a couple to conceive.

A baby may also be put at risk by one or more episodes of very heavy drinking — that is, if a woman drinks a large amount of absolute alcohol, about 3oz (three times the amounts listed above), over a few hours. If this happens in the first few weeks of pregnancy when the baby's organs are developing, there is an increased risk of damage, though the risk for the normally more abstemious woman remains low.

Some parents feel that since it has been proved that excess alcohol damages a baby, it is best to avoid it altogether, both before and during pregnancy. Giving up alcohol altogether can be part of taking some control over the pregnancy and cutting out all possible risks. For others, it seems reasonable to continue to drink small amounts during pregnancy since no study has ever shown that this has any adverse effect.

For advice and help with giving up alcohol, contact Alcohol Concern (see page 249 for the address).

## PRECONCEPTUAL CARE

Some parents decide to go further than the advice to maintain good general health and turn to one of the individuals or organisations that offer detailed advice on preconceptual care, especially on diet and dietary supplements and the avoidance of toxic (poisonous) substances. They find that the conviction and reassurance they are offered supports them through a difficult time. However, many researchers question the benefits of the kinds of strict regime recommended by some of the preconceptual care organisations, most of which have never been subjected to strict scientific trials. They also question the validity of some of these organisations' statistical claims to improve the rate of successful outcomes in pregnancy.

Each parent must decide for herself or himself about what will be supportive in another pregnancy. The approach of the preconceptual care organisations helps many parents and increases their sense of taking some control over the pregnancy. For others, their emphasis on individual parents' personal responsibility for the outcome of pregnancy is threatening. It can feel like blame in an area where most parents are only too ready to blame themselves, and can suggest certainty where there is little scientific evidence.*

*For a detailed discussion of the risks and benefits of drugs in and before pregnancy, including dietary supplements such as vitamins and minerals, medical drugs, alcohol, cigarettes and herbal and homeopathic remedies, see Judy Priest, *Drugs in Pregnancy and Childbirth* (London: Pandora, 1990).

## AVOIDING DANGEROUS ORGANISMS DURING PREGNANCY

Certain organisms which can exist in food and in the environment are known to cause late miscarriages, stillbirth and premature labour. Although cases in the UK and other developed countries are rare, many people feel that it is worth avoiding possible sources of these organisms during pregnancy. The main known dangerous organisms are listeria and toxoplasma gondii.

**Listeriosis** (see also page 191), caused by the bacteria listeria, is usually contracted from meat and dairy products — particularly some soft-ripened cheeses, cooked-chilled, ready-to-eat poultry, pâté and other cooked-chilled meals. The listeria bacteria is unusual in that it can multiply at 4°C, the temperature of many refrigerators. In the UK, the government recommends that pregnant women should not eat soft-ripened cheeses of the Brie, Camembert and blue-veined types, whether made from pasteurised or unpasteurised milk. Pregnant women should also take particular care to reheat cooked-chilled meals and ready-cooked poultry until it is piping hot right the way through.

In addition, the government in the UK recommends that everyone should take the following precautions to help prevent infection from listeria and other similar bacteria:

- Check that fridges are working properly and keep food really cold.
- Keep foods for as short a time as possible, follow storage instructions carefully and observe 'best by' and 'eat by' dates.
- Cook all poultry and meat products well. Reheat cooked-chilled meals thoroughly. Wash all salads, fruit and vegetables that will be eaten raw.
- Store raw foods and cheeses away from cooked foods in the fridge.
- Never reheat food more than once. Reheated food should be very hot all the way through.
- Allow foods that have been reheated in a microwave to stand as recommended by the oven manufacturers to ensure that they are well heated right through.
- Throw away left-over reheated food.

- Cool cooked food which is not to be eaten straight away as quickly as possible outside the fridge, then store it in the fridge.

**Rubella (German measles)** (see also page 192) Women can ask their GP for a test for rubella before they become pregnant. This will tell them whether or not they are immune to the disease. If they are not, they should be vaccinated and then avoid conceiving for three months.

**Toxoplasmosis** is a parasitic organism that can cause serious and fatal problems to a baby during pregnancy (see also page 193). The Toxoplasmosis Trust advises pregnant women to wear gloves when emptying cat litter trays and for gardening, especially if the soil might be contaminated with cat faeces; to wash their hands after emptying cat trays, gardening and handling raw meat; to avoid eating raw or undercooked meat; and to wash fruit and vegetables thoroughly.

Women can ask their GP for a test for toxoplasmosis before they become pregnant. This will tell them if they have had the disease and are therefore immune. Tests for toxoplasmosis can be carried out during pregnancy if an infection is suspected. If these confirm that the mother has had toxoplasmosis during the pregnancy, she can be treated with special antibiotics. Further tests may also be carried out, for example, cordocentesis (see Fetal blood sampling, page 144), to find out whether the baby has also been infected. If the baby is found to have been infected (which occurs in about 40 per cent of cases) stronger antibiotics will be given. These cannot reverse any damage that may already have been caused to the baby, but can significantly prevent further damage.

For more information about toxoplasmosis contact the Toxoplasmosis Trust (see page 247 for address).

## FEELINGS ABOUT A NEW PREGNANCY

For many bereaved parents a new pregnancy brings an upsetting mixture of emotions. The joy and hope they expect are often accompanied by anxiety about the new baby and intense sadness for the baby who died:

'All the sickness I had, backache, etc., were like medals to me when I was pregnant again. But the waiting and the worrying were terrible.'

Sometimes anxiety and renewed grief seem almost to overshadow any positive feelings. Gail gave birth to twin girls. The first was stillborn, the second was healthy and well. Six months later Gail was pregnant again:

'I'm terrified. Although I don't want to get rid of the pregnancy, I don't think I'm ready physically or emotionally. I feel so confused, so lucky to have one beautiful, healthy baby daughter but missing my other one, the other twin, so much. The thought of having another baby soon frightens me and brings back all the bad memories.'

Many parents find that their next pregnancy brings a new wave of sorrow for the baby who died. Maria's second child, Gerard, was stillborn. Six months into her next pregnancy, Maria found herself overwhelmed with grief and longing, and worried that she would not be able to love and care for her new baby in the way that she wanted:

'I want this new baby and so does my husband, but nothing can replace Gerard. Not a day goes by that I don't think about him. I'm scared that when I have this baby (although I'm really looking forward to its arrival), I might neglect it because the further on in pregnancy I get the more I find myself crying over Gerard, only nobody knows this, everybody thinks I'm all right. I'm scared of what my feelings will be for this baby and I'm scared of losing this baby. I feel so mixed up.'

Some women find themselves fantasizing that they are carrying again the baby who died. There is a need to 'undo' what happened before and to replay events, but this time with a happy ending. Gina's first baby, Peter, was stillborn. Her next pregnancy was filled with complex feelings and fantasies, which were resolved only when her new baby was born:

'Logically I knew that I would never have my baby back, although when I became pregnant again this didn't stop me day-dreaming and wishing I could swap the baby in my stomach for my "real" baby. She was always second best right up until she was born and then, well, I can't describe the emotion and absolute love I felt for her.'

Bereaved parents have lost their 'innocence' about pregnancy. They now know that babies can and do die and the devastating grief and pain that result. They know that they are embarking upon a hazardous process and can no longer take success for granted. Many parents feel that they and this new pregnancy are very vulnerable:

> 'Previously I'd always been eager for the confirmation of a positive test and rushed to tell family and friends. This time I knew myself I was pregnant — but just wanted to keep it quietly between my husband and myself for the first three months. I was happy — but not with a bubbly excitement — never again would I take for granted the straightforward birth of a healthy child.'

Janet P found the first few months of her fourth pregnancy pointless and unreal. After the death of her second child, Emma, and an early miscarriage, she had lost confidence in her ability to carry a pregnancy through to the delivery of a healthy baby:

> 'The midwife at the booking clinic asked me if I was going to breastfeed or bottle feed the new baby. That's a silly question, I thought, I'm not going to have a baby, so why does it matter how I'm going to feed it?'

For a few parents, there is a specific medical problem which means that there is a real medical risk of their pregnancy failing. Janet M lost seven babies due to rhesus disease. Like many women who know that they are obstetrically at high risk, she survived through each pregnancy by expecting failure:

> 'If you know that medically there's a high risk, you prepare yourself. You just stop expecting anything to come out of the pregnancy. What helped me to cope was that the doctors were absolutely straight with me. I knew that in my case it was very unlikely that I would succeed, I found out as much about rhesus disease as I could, I looked at my own medical notes, I labelled myself high risk and I let other people do the same. Some people found the fact that I didn't pretend very upsetting, a few people thought I was abnormal and found it frightening, but actually in my situation it was essential. I was being completely realistic.'

Many parents protect themselves against the pain that other people can cause, however unwittingly. Fiona S's first three babies were stillborn. When she became pregnant again she was very careful to make it clear to other people that the outcome of this pregnancy was not certain, so that she would not be caused unnecessary extra pain by unthinking questions and remarks if this baby also died:

> 'When people asked me, "When's it due?" I said, "Well, I haven't had a very good track record with babies, so if all goes well . . ." People actually respond very well if you say that to them, but I did protect myself all the way, I didn't buy anything or anything like that.'

Fiona's fourth and last baby was also stillborn.

Many bereaved parents find that one of their most important sources of support in another pregnancy is other bereaved parents. Often it feels as though these are the only people who understand what they are going through, and possibly the only people who are ready to listen sympathetically again and again to the sadness and anxiety stirred up by another pregnancy. One useful source of support may be a local self-help group for bereaved parents.

It can be very hard to cope with the day-to-day strain and anxiety of another pregnancy. Many parents find that the only way to get through is to take the pregnancy one step at a time. For Christa, in the pregnancy that followed the death of her twins, it helped to set a series of target stages, and to try to think no further than reaching the end of each stage:

> 'At my first antenatal visit to the GP I cried, at my first hospital visit I cried, and in between I felt strangely ambivalent yet convinced that I was going to have an early miscarriage. My thoughts went as far as getting through the first twelve weeks.
> 'At sixteen weeks I felt this baby move. This proved to be a small turning point, the baby was real and deserved to be loved and believed in. Part of me still looked back though, I couldn't afford the optimism.
> 'The next week was scan time again. Baby fine, it looked beautiful. Around this time I was convinced that I was going to go into premature labour again and set myself the target of getting to the twenty-fifth week which was the point at which disaster struck last time. One of the strangest things was trying to buy things for the baby. I would go into shops and try to buy something, just a pair of bootees, a bonnet, anything, just something to show faith. I couldn't do it. Some invisible force was stopping me.

'My next target was to get to Christmastime and thirty weeks. I knew that if the baby came then it would stand a good chance of survival. Christmas came and went with no relief from the worry, the worry just changed; now the baby would die *in utero* or be stillborn.'

Towards the end of the pregnancy Christa had another scan because of fears about the baby's growth:

'The day of the scan dawned. The minute the baby appeared on the screen I was asking "How big is it?" I was told to wait until all the measurements were done. Enough said that on the next day I was able to go out and spend a fortune on baby things and felt really excited for the first time. It was the release I needed.'

Christa's baby, Max, was born alive and well.

## ANTENATAL CARE

It can be very hard for parents to go back to the hospital where their baby died. Some choose to go to another hospital for their new pregnancy, though this is impossible if their local hospital is the only one in the area. But sometimes there is comfort in being back in a familiar place with staff who understand their circumstances and needs and are willing to give extra attention and care. Sallie's first child, James, was born prematurely at twenty-eight weeks gestation and lived for ten days:

'I had wonderful support from everyone throughout my next pregnancy, from midwives, social workers, doctors and, mainly, the consultant. People who had known me when James was alive for his brief time were all encouraging and supporting me. It was really terrific. A lot of people knew me by then and the hospital was practically my second home. The consultant took care of every single worry. Every unforeseen pain had a question mark over it. Was it abnormal? Or, worse, was it premature labour again? I needed him to explain it.'

The quality of antenatal care that bereaved parents receive in a subsequent pregnancy is extremely important. They need efficient and sympathetic care with opportunities to discuss and investigate, if necessary, any worries that they may have. They need to be able to feel confident in the professionals looking after them, and to know that their particular needs and anxieties are recognised, respected, and taken into account.

Many parents find additional scans or other tests helpful, even though, for some, they may not provide the reassurance that is so badly needed. Janet P had a very technological pregnancy with frequent tests and lots of explanation from the consultant in charge of her care. But although each test showed that all was well, she was never confident of the outcome of the pregnancy:

> 'Physically everything was fine and the baby was developing normally, but I was unable to accept this. At seventeen weeks I had a scan with a consultant radiologist. She told me everything was perfectly normal and I then realised that she could go on saying that until she was blue in the face, but, while I could accept that the baby was OK today, that did not mean it would be OK next week.'

Some parents, particularly those whose babies are known to be at high risk and who may therefore have a lot of medical intervention in their next pregnancy, can feel that they and their pregnancy are almost taken over by professionals. Janet M spent a good deal of time during her different pregnancies in a hospital which was a regional centre for women with high-risk pregnancies. Although the medical care and attention she received were excellent, she sometimes found the strain almost intolerable:

> 'The consultant was exceptional and involved us in everything, he shared everything with us, made us part of it all. But when he wasn't around it was easy to feel with some of the doctors that all they were interested in was your womb, and that you were just tagged on to it. I felt with some of the doctors as if my pregnancy belonged to them and I was doing it all for them. It became a challenge for them in its own right. In a way, I could accept that because, after all, we were all trying to achieve the same thing — a live healthy baby — but it could be very depersonalising sometimes.'

Like Janet, most parents find that, as well as high quality clinical care, they need to be fully informed about what is going on. They also need extra opportunities to talk to the professionals who are caring for them about their feelings as the pregnancy progresses, and particularly to discuss reactions that may surprise or upset them.

If parents have needs like these which are not being met, or any other problems with their care, it can help to get things out into the open and find someone at the hospital to talk to. Some parents arrange a special appointment to discuss what they feel about their antenatal care and the prospect of facing labour and delivery in the place where their baby died. Sometimes they also need to talk to someone about questions, anxieties and anger that may remain unresolved from their earlier experience, or about the care they are receiving now.

The most obvious person to talk to is usually the consultant, but some parents prefer to see the sister in charge of the antenatal clinic, their community midwife or another professional with whom they have a good relationship.

For Janet P. such a meeting was a turning point. Her daughter, Emma, was born prematurely and died of heart failure when she was six and a half weeks old. The post-mortem produced no specific cause for Emma's death, and Janet and her husband were left with many unanswered questions. During a later pregnancy, Janet's obstetrician arranged a meeting for her and her husband with a paediatrician from the special care baby unit:

'My husband and I had felt that there was a lack of communication between us and the medical staff, particularly after Emma died. This time we met a doctor who had recently joined the unit and therefore had not been part of the team caring for Emma. He looked through Emma's records, spoke to the staff and went through everything with us, patiently answering questions and never taking offence or feeling criticised by anything we said. He felt that her heart had been the key to all her problems, not prematurity, and that was reassuring as I had just had a trace done which showed that the new baby had a perfectly regular heartbeat.'

Some parents find that the experience of losing a baby has undermined their confidence and that they now find it particularly difficult to deal with health professionals. It may help to enlist some support, perhaps from a close friend or relative who can understand and share anxieties and problems but who is also objective in a way that parents themselves can never be.

Such a person might, for example, come regularly to hospital appointments to give moral support.

The tragedy of losing a baby can give parents the confidence to demand the care that they need in their next pregnancy. Following a stillbirth and then an early miscarriage, Cathy received little understanding or support from the professionals involved. During her next pregnancy, she wrote:

> 'I have found my doctor, local midwives and health visitor to be entirely uncommunicative, giving the impression that they have no sympathy or understanding of the trauma of stillbirth, or how deeply a baby can be missed. After Tim was stillborn my doctor's advice was "Don't upset yourself, you'll feel better soon." And the only communication I got from the community midwives at the time was a reminder to attend my antenatal classes! I have decided that the most positive action I can take in this new pregnancy, both for myself and for others who find themselves in my position, will be to try to explain my feelings to my doctor and to the professionals at the health centre. Perhaps if I spell out what support I needed after the stillbirth and the subsequent miscarriage, and the high level of understanding and support I would like to have in order to get through this pregnancy with the least anxiety possible, they might respond more to my needs.'

## ANTENATAL DIAGNOSIS

Parents may be offered extra investigations during another pregnancy, either to test for some special condition, or to help allay their own heightened anxieties and those of the people caring for them. Anything that can be done to give reassurance about the baby's well-being is likely to be welcome. Even so, antenatal diagnostic tests can be an ordeal, because they raise the possibility of another death, another loss. Parents may need a lot of support to help them face the tests, the waiting and the results.

A detailed explanation of the test and how it works should always be given beforehand. This should include what the test can and cannot diagnose, any risks involved in the test, how long the results will take to come through, how reliable they will be and what the options will be if it indicates that the baby is at risk or developing abnormally in some way.

In a small number of cases, diagnostic tests will show that the baby has a developmental abnormality. The nature of the abnormality and its severity must be explained clearly and sympathetically to the parents. When people are in a state of shock they are unlikely to absorb all that is said to them. It is helpful to confirm what was discussed in writing so that they can absorb the information slowly in the security of their own home. Parents may need two or three meetings to go over and discuss again what has been said to them.

If parents are faced with the very difficult decision of whether to terminate the pregnancy, they need clear information, understanding care, and sympathetic, informed support from the professionals who are caring for them. They also need privacy, both when they are seeing professionals and when they are alone together, information about how the termination would be carried out, including pain relief, and as much time as they wish to think about their decision. They need to be reassured that, if they decide on a termination, they will be supported and cared for physically and emotionally, and that their baby's body will be treated with dignity and respect. After the termination they may wish to see and hold their baby, to hold some form of funeral or other ceremony, and to create a physical memorial for their baby to which they can return in years to come.

Some parents whose baby is found to have an abnormality which will inevitably be fatal or severely handicapping, choose not to terminate the pregnancy, but to wait and let nature take its course. They may be able to use the remaining weeks of the pregnancy to begin to come to terms with what this baby will mean to them and how they will manage. If the baby is unlikely to live for more than a few hours or days after birth, they may wish to think about ways in which they can honour and celebrate their baby's life, however short, and to plan a funeral and other memorials.

Whatever decision the parents take, everyone involved in their care from this point on must be aware of their situation and provide a high level of care and support. Parents who are considering the possibility of terminating a pregnancy and would like information and support, may like to contact Support After Termination For Abnormality (SATFA), see page 245 for the address.

## Tests that may be used during pregnancy

**Ultrasound scans** These use high frequency sound waves to create a picture of the baby in the womb. A transducer is passed backwards and forwards over the mother's abdomen; this beams sound waves through the abdomen into the womb. The sound waves bounce back off the baby and are translated into a picture on a screen.

Ultrasound scans can be used:

- to check that the baby is growing and developing normally
- to check that the baby's heart is beating and that he or she is still alive
- to check the baby's age (this is most reliable before twenty weeks gestation)
- to find the baby's position and the position of the placenta
- to help other diagnostic procedures such as amniocentesis and chorion villus sampling
- to find out if there is more than one baby
- to check the shape of the womb and detect growths such as fibroids
- to help detect some structural abnormalities, including some neural tube defects and, sometimes, abnormalities in the heart, kidney, bowel and other organs. A skilled ultrasonographer can spot most structural abnormalities on a scan. If a structural abnormality is feared or suspected, parents may be referred to a specialist ultrasound unit for further more detailed scanning.

Many bereaved parents who are anxious about the development and well-being of a subsequent baby find the sight of a living, healthy baby on the screen extremely reassuring. But a scan can also be very worrying. For parents whose previous baby was stillborn or died shortly after birth, their last scan may have been the moment when they finally realised that the baby had died or could not live. Many bereaved parents experience strong and often confused emotions at the sight of their new baby on the screen.

The way the scan is managed is very important. Most women wish to have someone of their choice accompanying them — their partner, a relative or a close friend. The picture on the screen is usually difficult to interpret and needs to be explained, at least in general terms. In some hospitals scans are carried out by technicians who may not be permitted to tell the parents what they see on the screen. For parents who are under the additional strain of an earlier bereavement or who have particular reason to fear bad news, this can be very hard.

In this situation a scan should, wherever possible, be carried out by a professional who can interpret and explain the findings to the parents on the spot. When the scan is booked parents may wish to check what arrangements are planned and to stress the importance of having someone present who can explain it to them straightaway. If this is really not possible, parents should be told who will give them the information and how long they will have to wait. During the scan, they should be supported and encouraged to ask any questions about the scan findings.

**Alpha-feto protein test** This is a blood test to find out how much alpha-fetoprotein (AFP) from the baby is in the mother's blood. AFP is a protein made in the baby's liver and not found in adults. If the baby's skin is broken, for example by an open neural tube defect (see page 205) or an abnormality in the baby's abdominal wall, or if the baby has a kidney abnormality, additional AFP may pass into the amniotic fluid and eventually into the mother's blood where it can be detected. Over 80 per cent of cases of anencephaly and over 70 per cent of cases of open neural tube defects can be detected by an AFP test.

There is also a link between lower than average levels of AFP and Down's syndrome. However, only 20 to 30 per cent of babies with Down's syndrome will be detected by an AFP test (see also Bart's blood test below).

A blood test for AFP is usually offered at between sixteen and eighteen weeks and the results take a few days to come. It is very important to do the test at the right point of gestation since the level of AFP in the mother's blood increases as the pregnancy continues; if the test is done later it might give a misleading result.

A raised AFP level does not always mean that the baby has one of the abnormalities listed above. It can mean that there are two or more babies or, since a baby makes larger quantities of AFP as the pregnancy progresses, that the pregnancy is further on than was thought. A low level of AFP does not always indicate Down's syndrome. But if a raised or low level of AFP is found the mother may be offered a second AFP test. Amniocentesis (see below) or ultrasound (see above) will then be offered to confirm the diagnosis.

**Bart's blood test** This is a blood test that can help detect Down's syndrome in a baby in the womb. At present it is only available in a few specialist centres. Blood from the mother is tested for three factors: alpha-feto protein from the baby (see above) and two hormones produced mainly by the placenta — oestriol and Beta HCG (Human Chorionic Gonadotrophin). The level of these, calculated with the mother's age and the length of the pregnancy, can indicate the level of risk that the baby has Down's syndrome. If the risk is greater than one in 200, the parents will be offered amniocentesis (see below). The Bart's blood test can detect between 40 and 60 per cent of babies with Down's syndrome.

**Amniocentesis** This involves inserting a fine needle through the wall of the mother's abdomen and into her womb to draw off a sample of the amniotic fluid (liquor) which surrounds the baby. The position of the baby and the placenta are checked on ultrasound scan during the procedure, so that they are not damaged by the needle. Amniocentesis is normally carried out at about sixteen to eighteen weeks gestation.

Amniotic fluid contains both chemicals and cells from the baby. The chemicals can be tested immediately but the cells must be grown (cultured) for about three weeks to produce enough for testing.

Tests can show:

- abnormal chromosomes which may indicate developmental abnormalities such as Edwards' syndrome, Patau's syndrome or Down's syndrome (see pages 202–5)
- genes which may indicate an inherited disease such as sickle cell disease (see page 199) or thalassaemia (see page 218)
- the sex of the baby
- rhesus disease (see page 209)
- enzyme levels, to see whether the baby has a metabolic disorder, such as Tay-Sachs disease.

Although amniocentesis is a very useful diagnostic tool, it has several disadvantages. At present about one in every 200 amniocentesis tests causes a miscarriage. If there is a raised APF level in the amniotic fluid the risk of miscarriage seems to be higher, though it is not clear whether this is linked with the amniocentesis. Some parents feel that the risk of a miscarriage is too high. For others, it is very important to know as soon as possible whether their new baby has a major developmental abnormality.

Amniocentesis can only be carried out between sixteen and eighteen weeks and the cells then take two to three weeks to culture, so the decision whether to terminate the pregnancy if the baby is affected must be taken very late. In about 2 per cent of cases the cells do not culture and the amniocentesis has to be repeated, causing further delays.

**Chorionic villus sampling (CVS)** This is a newer technique than amniocentesis and is at present only available in a few hospitals. Parents should be referred to a specialist centre by their own obstetrician if necessary. CVS can be carried out between the eighth and eleventh weeks of pregnancy to test for certain inherited diseases including sickle cell disease (see page 199) and thalassaemia (see page 218), for most chromosomal abnormalities, such as Edwards' syndrome, Patau's syndrome and Down's syndrome (see pages 202–5), and for metabolic disorders, such as Tay-Sachs disease. It cannot diagnose neural tube defects.

A very fine tube is passed into the mother's womb either through her abdomen or through her vagina. An ultrasound scan is used to guide the tube to the chorionic villi, the beginnings of the placenta, and a tiny sample of the villi is sucked out and removed. Because the chorionic villi are developed from the original fertilised egg, the cells in the sample can give information about the baby's genetic make-up. The cells are then grown (cultured) for two or three weeks to produce enough for testing, though in the case of certain rare conditions the results may take longer to come through.

The major advantage of CVS is that it can be done relatively early in pregnancy. This means that if the test shows that the baby has severe developmental or other problems, and the parents decide to terminate the pregnancy, this can be done at a much earlier stage than is possible after amniocentesis.

However, CVS also has certain known disadvantages. One is that at present the rate of miscarriage following CVS is higher than that following amniocentesis (about 4 in every 100 cases compared with about 2 in every 100), though it is likely that since CVS is carried out earlier in pregnancy some of these pregnancies would always have gone on to miscarry anyway. A second, and linked, known disadvantage is that sometimes severe chromosomal abnormalities are diagnosed and medical terminations carried out on pregnancies that would have ended naturally in the next few weeks.

Since CVS is a new and important technique large research studies are currently underway to see whether it has other disadvantages. The full picture will not be clear until the findings of these studies emerge. As with all diagnostic procedures, it is important that parents who are considering CVS are fully informed about the known advantages and disadvantages before deciding whether to go ahead.

**Fetal blood sampling** Samples of the baby's blood (fetal blood) can be used to detect many chromosomal abnormalities (see pages 202–5) and toxoplasmosis (see page 193). They can be used to diagnose sickle cell disease (see page 199) and thalassaemia (see page 218), though chorionic villi sampling (see above) is generally preferable since it can be done earlier in pregnancy. Fetal blood samples can also be used to assess the degree of anaemia in a baby with rhesus disease (see page 209).

Fetal blood sampling can be carried out at any time after about eighteen weeks of pregnancy, but the precise timing of each test depends on what is being looked for. The sample of fetal blood is usually taken from a blood vessel in the umbilical cord: this is known as cordocentesis. If the baby's position in the womb makes this impossible the blood may be taken from a large vein in the baby's abdomen. A fine needle is injected through the wall of the mother's abdomen and a small sample of blood drawn off. Ultrasound is used so that the doctor can guide the needle accurately.

The results of the blood tests normally take about a week to come through though there may be some delay if the samples have to be sent off to specialist laboratories. Fetal blood sampling is thought to cause a miscarriage in about one in every 100 cases, though this rate increases if the baby is already ill or weak.

Fetal blood sampling is at present carried out in only a few specialist centres. Parents should be referred to a specialist centre by their own obstetrician if necessary.

**Other tests** Other tests may be carried out during the pregnancy to check on the baby's health. These may include, for example, serial ultrasound scans to check that the baby is growing at the right rate, fetal heart rate traces, and Doppler blood flow studies which check the health of the placenta and the baby.

## PREPARING FOR ANOTHER DELIVERY

The prospect of another delivery is often frightening. Inevitably, it brings back painful memories and fears. Although many parents find it hard to look ahead to the birth because it seems to be tempting fate, making plans and discussing how they would like the birth to be handled can also calm fears and overcome worries. Some parents find it helpful to talk to a sympathetic and understanding doctor or midwife about what happened last time, to talk through their fears about the coming birth, and to discuss how they would like this delivery managed, what they hope for and what they want to prepare for that is either the same or different.

This is not just a matter of planning the delivery in order to reduce medical risk. Other considerations may also be important. For example, parents may want (or not want) to be in the same delivery room as before, they may want particular people with them, they may want certain practical details to be different or the same. They may have strong feelings about pain relief and other interventions and about how they would like the labour to be managed generally. They may want to discuss the possibility of urgent medical intervention being necessary and how they would like this handled. Some women may want their partners to be with them the whole time, no matter what happens. Both parents may feel that it is important that they should be kept fully informed throughout the labour and be warned in advance of any intervention the professionals are considering. Some parents may want the baby to be handed to them as soon as possible. Others may want any essential checks to be carried out on the baby first, so that they can be fully reassured that this time all is well.

June and Greg's first son, Philip, was stillborn. About a year later June became pregnant again. After an anxious pregnancy the time came for their second baby to be born. June was going to have another caesarean, again under epidural, and welcomed the fact that she would be at the same hospital with the same consultant and anaesthetist:

'It may seem strange that this felt good, because of course the associations with last time were very strong. I know Greg found it difficult but it was very important to me. I didn't want to forget Philip at this point — and indeed one of the hardest things to cope with in the coming days was the way in which most people did forget him.'

But there was one detail which June did want to be different. Philip had been wrapped in a blue blanket, so June asked the midwife if the new baby, whatever its sex, could have a pink blanket:

'I have so little to remember Philip by, and his blanket somehow had to be his alone.'

June's emotions at this birth were very different from those she had felt when Philip was born, but she knew that this difference did not mean that she would love her new baby, Richard, any less. From the moment of his birth she was content to trust her feelings and to accept the difference:

'Just as I'd felt stunned on first learning of Philip's death, whereas Greg had been quite overcome, so we seemed to play similar reactions to this birth. I hardly registered the baby's first cry. Greg, on the other hand, wept tears of joy and relief. I was moved by that more than anything.

'In a while, Greg took Richard and cuddled him. He told me later that he felt then the intense emotion which I had anticipated feeling myself. I think I had imagined I would re-experience the overwhelming rush of love I'd known when I stroked Philip's downy head and held him against my body, knowing that this was the first and last time I'd be with him. But with his brother, Richard, it was different, this first meeting. And the difference was good. As I gazed at this tiny creature, so weak and yet so strong, I knew that very soon he would be getting a firm grip on my heart and on my life.'

# 6 Another Baby

For many parents the birth of a new baby fulfills all their hopes. They grow to love their new baby and to regain their confidence as parents. Some of the painful memories and anxieties that still remain begin to heal, so that the baby who died is remembered with enduring love and with less distress:

> 'Before Melanie was born I was afraid of having a reaction, but she just fitted into our lives from day one. She was Melanie, her own self, our third child and part of our life. Despite the stress of the pregnancy she is the happiest, most delightful baby, and has a big beaming smile for which you forgive her everything.
>
> 'From the time Melanie was three to four months old I began to accept that she was a perfectly normal baby. I had got over the initial tiredness and an attack of the flu, Christmas, and the anniversaries of Emma's birth and death. The doctor at the hospital pronounced us "normal parents again". It was only then that I realised how difficult I'd been — that "normal" people didn't go round bursting into tears, and how chronically tired I'd been, even before I got pregnant with Melanie. It was like emerging from a dark tunnel into the warm sunlight.'

But often it takes time for all this to happen. For very many parents the first weeks and months of their new baby's life are also filled with pain and confusion, and with renewed sorrow for the baby they have lost. Gina's first baby, Peter, was stillborn. Throughout her next pregnancy she felt that no other baby could ever be as perfect or as important to her as he was. When her daughter, Florence, was born she found herself overwhelmed by the absolute love she felt for her, but also torn by a painful new understanding of what she had lost:

> 'My only difficulty was that I felt greedy. I knew full well that I wouldn't have had Florence if Peter had lived but now I wanted both of them. I was in complete turmoil. I had never realised I could love

a baby as much as I loved Florence and now I realised what I had been missing out on. I should have had two babies, not one.'

Sometimes the sorrow which returns at the birth of another baby can even overwhelm parents' feelings of happiness and love for the new baby. Although this stage passes, they may at first feel guilty that they are not loving their new baby as they feel they should, or anxious that they will never be able to be 'normal' loving parents. Dawn's first baby, Cara, was stillborn. A few weeks later she became pregnant again, and after a difficult pregnancy gave birth to her second daughter, Kirsty. Kirsty's birth reawakened all Dawn's longing and unresolved grief for Cara and she found herself thinking more about Cara than about Kirsty:

'While I was pregnant with Kirsty I didn't think too much about Cara. I was more concerned about my health and my unborn child. But now, all I seem to think about is Cara, even though I have a wonderful baby who is alive. I keep thinking if Kirsty looks like Cara and there are many other things I try and compare.

'Everything is so fresh in my mind but everyone else seems to have forgotten. I still feel so guilty about Cara's death. No one else ever talks about her but I seem to mention her all the time.'

It is understandable if the experience of giving birth and holding a newborn baby once again triggers memories and a flood of new grief. But many parents are quite unprepared for what may, on the surface, seem a perverse reaction to the birth. Sallie felt that if she had had some warning and the chance to talk about possible reactions beforehand, she might have found her feelings less difficult to cope with. Her first child, James, lived for ten days. The birth of her second son, John, brought back painful memories of James's birth and short life:

'At first when John was born, I felt this tremendous happiness, but I remember having very nearly a complete breakdown about three days later, because it had all brought back James's birth. It was an extraordinary time of feeling completely up in the air but also devastated with grief for James. And everybody was saying, "Isn't this wonderful, you must be over the moon," and I felt, "My God! How can I cope?" I was weeping buckets. And I was quite cross that nobody had warned me that I might feel anything like that. I might have found it easier to cope with.'

Rosalind, whose baby, Georgia, was stillborn, had been warned she might find the first few weeks and months of her new baby's life difficult. But her longing for another baby was so great that she could not believe that this would be true for her:

'I got pregnant again reasonably quickly, and thought I was OK. I was still grieving for Georgia, but there was hope again, a baby growing inside me. I never realised that I thought it was Georgia, a second chance to have her properly, so I never prepared myself for the fact that I was having a different baby. She was induced two weeks early to avoid another placental abruption, so the labour felt artificial and unreal. It was only ten and a half months after Georgia died and I was at a very low ebb. We were in the delivery room next door to where I'd been when I had Georgia, and I felt miles away from everyone.

'Molly was tiny, and frail, and born in distress and with the cord round her neck tightly, twice. The shock of nearly losing her too was too much and I felt no exhilaration, no joy, just terribly sad and tired. She was a pretty, sweet baby and I held her but felt nothing really. I wanted my real baby back.

'All the grief I'd kept bottled up while I was pregnant came pouring out, and didn't stop for three months. I was inundated with cards and flowers and presents and visitors wanting to share in my joy, but I didn't feel any, just pity for Georgia that she'd missed out on all this, and for Molly because I couldn't feel enough for her.

'I wasn't me for a while. I threw Tom out for a bit, I screamed at the other kids, and I cried, all day, every day. I don't really know why things improved, but they did, slowly. Molly stopped being a tiny baby and grew into an assertive and funny little girl, no longer to be confused with her sister. All the right feelings turned up in due course, and the other children adore her too. In some ways she's a special favourite, maybe because we had to work hard at our relationship, and she *has* been the comfort everyone expected — it just wasn't immediate.'

Many parents find that it takes time and conscious effort to develop love for their new baby, and perhaps to get over the disappointment that this baby is not the one who died, nor the almost identical 'replacement' they had dreamed about:

'John and I really had to work hard at loving our new baby boy. We had both wanted a girl to replace our little Julie. It seemed to take weeks before a loving bond came.'

Parents who feel that the survival of their new baby is at particular risk may, consciously or unconsciously, shut off their emotions during the pregnancy. They may at first feel little for the new baby, and it may take time for a relationship to develop:

> 'I felt cold and detached as though she wasn't mine — even a cry for food meant little. I think on reflection that having switched off for nine months, just in case, I had done too good a job and this continued well after her birth. I never spoke about it, with everyone around us so happy. How would they understand that this baby meant little to me? She wasn't the one who had died and she wouldn't replace her. I felt a total disinterest in her for some time.'

It can be impossibly hard for parents who have been bereaved to tell anyone about the sorrow and stress they are experiencing in the months after the birth of another baby. There is often tremendous pressure to be, or at least to seem to be, happy. Even close family and friends may be unable to accept parents' sadness and confused feelings. They may think that the time for mourning is now over and that for parents to continue to talk about the baby who died and to grieve for him or her is undesirable and unhealthy. Because witnessing other people's distress can be so painful, they may want the parents to 'forget' the baby who died and to be happy with the one they have.

But every child, every baby, is a different and unique person. Although some of the longing for a baby to love and hold may be taken away with a new birth, the baby who died does not matter any less, and is in no way replaced by a new baby:

> 'People told us that having Eleanor would lessen the pain of losing Bethan — but it hasn't. We both still cry for the child we had come to love but never knew, and her birthday was awful although I had a little one to cuddle all day.
>
> 'It is funny how other people see us as a young couple with a baby, whereas we feel we are a family that will never be complete.'

After the birth of her daughter, Becky, Fiona L also found it hard to cope with other people's assumptions that she should now feel happy again. Knowing that people around her expected her to be happy, and feeling guilty that she had caused them worry and distress in the past, she felt she could not tell them about her real feelings:

'All the time it was as though I was watching myself and just *saying* all the right things. People gave me lovely presents for the baby and I wrote all my thank-you letters and did everything I was supposed to, but inside I was battling just to get through the days.

'I tried to tell a few people outside the family but nobody really listened. And how *could* I tell family and friends I still felt so miserable? I just wanted them to be happy and I wanted to release them from the grief I had initially caused. So here I was, unable to acknowledge my despair and trying to be "normal". I desperately needed help. I suppose I could have done with bereavement counselling but I couldn't ask for it, I couldn't *say* how terrible things were. If someone had laid it on for me I would have taken it, but I couldn't ask.'

On top of her grief for her first baby, Fiona found herself up against the difficulties almost all mothers of young babies face. She had had little previous experience of small babies and the stress and exhaustion of motherhood came as a shock to her. She struggled through the first year of Becky's life, feeling extremely depressed and unable to cope:

'This was my first baby to care for and I didn't know just how hard it is normally to look after a small baby. I think I was suffering from both postnatal depression and still grieving the death of my first baby.

'Nobody ever seemed to have any idea of what I was going through. Nobody ever said, "It must be hard for you now you've got another baby." But for the first year of Becky's life I struggled to "cope". I wish somebody had said something to me and helped me realise that this was normal, if not OK.'

Few parents ever admit, even to each other, the difficulty and stress that they sometimes feel with a small baby. Yet all parents find the reality of parenting difficult, at times almost unbearably so, even without the pressures and strains of an earlier bereavement. If bereavement has also affected parents' confidence in themselves, they can easily assume that they are in some way at fault when things are difficult. Having mourned the baby who died with such pain, and waited with such hope and anxiety for the arrival of the new baby, how can they be less than deliriously happy?:

'Now that I had got my baby, my heart's desire, how could I tell anybody how miserable I was?'

It is important that bereaved parents find a way to express the whole range of their experience and feelings about their new baby and do not feel forced all the time to put on a good front. Janet P, whose daughter, Emma, died six and a half weeks before her birth, was aware of the pressure to do this when she wrote, a few days after her daughter, Melanie, was born alive and well:

> 'I do wonder how I will react to this new baby and how I will feel towards it when things are rough, at 3 o'clock in the morning, or at teatime. Will I be expected to be so grateful for having a baby that I should cheerfully suffer all inconvenience? Or will I be allowed to be fed up like other mums?'

Fears and worries that are not expressed can cause unnecessary extra pain and difficulty to parents who have already had enough to cope with. And the unexpected turmoil of emotions that follows the birth of their new baby may be eased if parents can find an understanding person to talk to. Some parents find their health visitor, GP or another professional helpful at this point. Others find support from other parents who have experienced the loss of a baby and who can offer the understanding that often no one else can. Gina telephoned the Stillbirth and Neonatal Death Society (SANDS) and was able to talk about her feelings over the phone. She then made contact with her local SANDS group and got to know other bereaved parents in her area:

> 'I spent the first six weeks of my daughter's life feeling both ecstatically happy at my good fortune and sad at the same time. It was during this time that I contacted SANDS for the first time. I had wanted to on many occasions but had never felt able to pick up the phone. I took the plunge eventually because I did not anticipate the renewal of grief, and missing my son so much.'

Joanne and Jeremy, whose son, Jason, died in special care eleven days after his birth, were helped after his death by a bereavement counsellor from the hospital. She continued to support them during their next pregnancy and for some time after the birth of their daughter, Francesca:

> 'When Francesca was born healthy and normal Jeremy and I were over the moon, but we had no idea how great would be the rekindling of

grief over Jason. We felt relieved that our new baby was a girl because she looked exactly like her brother and though devoted to her, we were torn apart with longing for our dead baby. Why, oh why, had he been denied life when she was alive and kicking? How could it have happened? Why wasn't Jason with us too? We desperately needed to talk our emotions through with someone who would listen and understand. It was vital to me that the feelings of guilt I had about being low and depressed after such a happy event were accepted. The counsellor reassured us that we were behaving quite normally by being desperate and sad after what we had been through.

'We were able finally to understand that only now as our second child was born could we "let go" some more of our grief for our first baby. Now that we had a baby to keep, to hold, to nurture, only now did we know the full extent of what we had lost.'

Parents who have been bereaved may find that the anxiety they felt during the next pregnancy continues after their baby is born. They now know very well how precious and also how fragile life is and they can find it very hard to believe that their new baby is safe. For many parents this heightened anxiety continues for many years. Jeanne, who had three stillborn daughters, feels that her special anxiety and concern for her son has become part of her life:

'We both feel we are fussier parents because of our losses. While he was a baby our son was checked constantly while he slept, blissfully unaware of our hovering. I still pop in to check him at night and said to a friend, "I'll probably still do that when he's seventeen and his girlfriend throws me out!" Any minor cough or cold is thought to be major, any childhood illness fraught with possible complications. But we can and do cope. We do not rush to the doctor with every sneeze; we are just aware of our feelings and failings. I would dearly love to be less controlled and controlling. Only time will tell how we have fared.'

For almost all parents, the loss of a baby also leaves a lasting sadness and a special and heightened sensitivity which the birth of another baby may never completely heal. Looking back, nine years after the death of her first son, and now with two more children, Fiona L is aware that although she has now come to accept her loss, she still carries with her the special vulnerability of those who have lost a child:

'Nine years on I am still only realising what an effect losing my first child had on me. As I begin to feel more content with life and more (though not completely) tolerant of being an imperfect mother, I realise how hard this time has been. I do feel I have come to terms with my loss to a great extent. A crack remains and can still open up — at times unexpectedly — but the emptiness inside has been filled.'

For almost all parents the arrival of a new baby triggers a period of acute renewed grief and pain. But it also begins, in time, a new phase of healing and comfort. Although they will never be the same again, and in many ways would not want to be, they can begin to feel again some connection with the real world and to invest hope and energy in the future.

# 7 Looking Back

In Chapter 1, parents told their own stories; in this chapter, those parents look back to the time of their baby's death and tell what has happened to them since.

## ANGELA

**Angela's daughter, Suzanne, died twenty-eight hours after she was born. Her story is on page 11. Angela already had two sons at the time, Daniel, then aged 8, and Matthew, aged 5. Her account of what happened after Suzanne's death falls into two parts. The first part looks back about eighteen months after Suzanne died.**

Five months after Suzanne died I found out that I was pregnant again. I was elated and the difference it made to me was incredible. I felt slightly happy again, despite the pain and aching for Suzanne. But at eight weeks this baby miscarried and I came home from hospital once again to face the pram, etc., that had now lost two babies.

I felt absolutely nothing, and at the same time so damned angry. I didn't know what to do, where to go, what to think. I felt a failure and inadequate as a woman. People said things like 'Oh, it was too early after Suzanne's death,' 'Never mind, it was probably for the best,' 'It's nature's way' and 'It's not as bad as losing Suzanne — you were only seven weeks.' My God, how could they say those things? Of course it wasn't as bad as losing Suzanne, but I loved and wanted that baby, to me it was a baby, not a fetus or a lump, but my baby. I really hoped it would be the miracle that Suzanne could not be.

My mind just kept saying, will somebody please, please help me. I felt lost, lonely and afraid. There had to be a limit to how much I could take and emotionally I think I'd had enough. Just after the miscarriage, when I was waiting to go into theatre, I prayed I'd die, I just couldn't go on. I knew I'd got Alan and the boys, but at the same time my body and my arms cried out for my babies.

Soon after the miscarriage we moved house. The house was in a poor condition so I threw myself into that, and I also got a part-time job. It was only relief work but it was something to do and the extra money was nice. I also went to my GP who put me on a preconceptual course of vitamins, etc., and I decided to lose some weight. The vitamins and weight loss were my idea, and my GP was happy to help. I was determined to get myself physically fit and emotionally stable, so that I'd done everything I possibly could to be prepared and carry a baby next time. Nothing and no one could make up for the babies I had lost, but I felt I had to go on and try again in the hope that happiness would be ours again.

I became pregnant quite soon. In myself I felt very well, sometimes sickly, but confident that this time everything would be OK. The time before I knew from the moment I thought I was pregnant that I was going to lose it. I don't know why I felt that but I did.

As Suzanne's first birthday approached, I found things increasingly difficult: I couldn't believe where the year had gone and I missed her terribly. Some days I was fine and confident about the next baby, but other days were completely awful. I found it hard to visualise holding and keeping another baby. Also, being pregnant again was difficult. I was glad I was, but all the waiting, wondering, hoping and feeling so ill again just seemed too much.

Dale Alexander was born sixteen months after Suzanne's death. The first forty-eight hours after he was born were the worst we had to endure. We kept a constant check on him. The medical staff took test after test, and he was under the same paediatrician who was with Suzanne when she died. All the tests were negative, but he did become jaundiced after two days and had phototherapy for nearly three days, so we left hospital when he was six days old.

I can't begin to tell you what it was like, dressing him in his own clothes and bringing him home. I felt so pleased and proud, but so sad at the same time that I never brought Suzanne home. I spent a great deal of time crying when I bathed him and did all the things you do with a baby, because it made me realise just what I'd missed with Suzanne, and how only a year before I was pretending in my mind that she was here and that I was actually doing things with her.

Don't misunderstand me, we love Dale with all our hearts — he is so special and such a beautiful, contented baby. We just wish that Suzanne was here to complete our happiness.

**Six months after Dale's birth, Angela became pregnant again and went on to have another son, Liam. A few weeks after Liam's birth, Angela wrote this account.**

It is now just over two and a half years since Suzanne died and so much has happened and the time has gone so quickly. We now have four sons, Daniel and Matthew, and Dale and Liam, who were born after Suzanne's death.

I always say that Dale gave me back my life. I had needed a baby so desperately, to hold and to love and to care for. I'm not saying it was easy. The pregnancy was a worry all the way through and after the birth the first two days were a nightmare, worrying and watching for any little thing. I had felt that the first day would be the worst, but it was not to be because once at home I continually worried about cot death. I felt sure he was going to die at some point, so I made the most of every minute, holding him, loving him and telling him just what I felt. I cried with him, laughed with him and slowly rebuilt my life to some degree.

I can look back now and see how much I've changed and how much stronger I am and, I hope, a better person than I was, more sensitive and caring, more patient and not materialistic. Life is for living and loving, and a family with love is so special and something to be treasured. I hope my children too are benefiting from what I've learnt. I suppose everyone says the same thing — why does it take a tragedy to learn something?

Finding out I was pregnant again with Liam was a shock. Everyone 'hoped it would be a girl'; they felt it would make everything OK, even make up for Suzanne's death. But I knew it wouldn't and no one could ever replace her or be the dreams and hopes we'd had for her. Of course Liam wasn't a girl and then everyone felt sorry for us, thinking we were disappointed, but we weren't at all. I found I was almost going overboard about how thrilled I was, to show people that I wasn't bothered, but even that backfired because they thought I was being 'very brave'! I simply couldn't win. Now I just act myself and don't care what they think. I know that we're happy and that's all that matters, isn't it?

Liam is a beautiful child, all our boys are, and Dale and Liam are in particular; and they are very special because we are now aware as we never were before how precious each pregnancy and new life is. I suppose I think about Suzanne more because Liam is our last child — we won't be having any more — and that our family is not complete without her. But from the minute she died our family was never going to be complete again, was it?

Life is very hectic but I enjoy it very much and looking back, I wouldn't change a thing. Of course I wouldn't want Suzanne to have died, but I would still want Dale and Liam and feel very much that they have enriched our lives through Suzanne's death.

I miss her still so very much and still have times of great sadness, longing to hold her and see her again, to tell her all the things that I couldn't tell her in her short life, to show her her brothers and her daddy and all the people who loved her so much before and after her birth, whose hearts were broken, as ours were, when she died. The times I've sat and wondered why, and I still don't know. I don't think we will until we meet again when my life is over. But all I can say is that I loved her and lost her and I'm glad that I held her and kissed her and showed her to friends and family, and that those twenty-eight hours with her were probably the most precious memories I have, and no one can take them away. She was and always will be our special little girl.

## ANN

**Ann tells the story of her son Christopher's stillbirth on page 13. Here she tells about the five years since his death.**

After the death of Christopher, my life changed. I come from a very close family background — there is only myself and one sister, and my husband is an only child. Children were important to us and the stillbirth affected us all extremely badly. At the time my sister was also pregnant with her first baby. She was due around Christmas, so in August when we lost Christopher she was about five months pregnant. It was a very traumatic time for us all, especially my poor mother who felt torn between her feelings for both of us. My sister was admitted to hospital in November with placenta praevia and was kept in until her baby, Emma, was born by section in early December. I hated visiting the hospital with all the other pregnant women and babies, but made myself face up to it.

I had left my job the June before Christopher was born and had not kept it open. I felt absolutely useless in every way. But I was finally offered a part-time job with the same firm, which suited me fine as I really wanted to get pregnant again straight away. This didn't happen. In fact, I had a lot of problems with heavy bleeding and was admitted to hospital for investigation under anaesthetic. Waking up from the operation was awful, I really felt at my lowest. I had lots of further tests and nobody seemed to know why I wasn't getting pregnant again. I was convinced I would never have any children.

The next year things went from bad to worse. I was still not pregnant and seeing my sister with her baby was upsetting. My best friend had also had her first baby just before Christopher, and it seemed that everyone everywhere was pregnant and having babies easily.

During the spring my dear mother became ill and in June she passed away. This was the worst time of my whole life. I saw her in the chapel of rest on my twenty-eighth birthday and just could not believe that in less than one year I had lost this beautiful person who had given me life on that same day all those years before, and that I myself had created a new life that was then so cruelly taken away from me. Why was I the one left? I cannot explain all my feelings on that day. I had never really experienced death before and, in such a short space of time, I had to face up to the death of both my mother and a child. At my mother's funeral, everyone talked of her life and its purpose, which made me feel more isolated. What purpose did Christopher have in life? It seemed to me that nobody really knew how I felt. My grief was so intense that looking back I really don't know what pulled me through.

I think it was then that I gained an extra inner strength from somewhere: I became determined not to waste my life. In a peculiar way, my mother's death helped me to come to terms with all that had happened and made me decide to make a fresh start. With my husband's help and support, I changed specialists and started to have all the tests again. I was determined to find out why I had not become pregnant and decided that if we couldn't have any more then we would do something useful with our lives and not waste any more time.

From that point, things moved quickly. The consultant found out that we were 'hostile' to each other, that we were incompatible but not totally infertile. He put me on a fertility drug, and also did a laparoscopy. Within the first month and the first course of tablets, I missed a period. On 26 June, exactly twelve months to the day since my mother's death, I found myself in the same hospital complex where I had watched my mother die, waiting for the results of a pregnancy test. It was positive! On that day of all days, it was incredible.

The pregnancy was very traumatic emotionally. At nine weeks and again at twelve I was admitted to hospital with heavy bleeding. On each occasion I had scans which to my surprise showed a heartbeat. I couldn't believe it was possible to lose so much blood and for everything to be normal. The second time it happened was just before what would have been Christopher's second birthday and this made me convinced that I would miscarry on that day. The anxiety was enormous. It was impossible for me to believe that things wouldn't go wrong.

At about six months, I started to get anxious about the baby's movements. This was the only indication for me with Christopher and the memories of that awful day when I was willing him to move kept coming back to me. I found myself awake at night terrified if the baby was still. The hospital were very good and said that if ever I was the least bit worried to go and they would put me on the monitor. So on two or three occasions I rang up and went for reassurance.

By the time I was about thirty-eight weeks, the specialist said that if I wanted he would induce the labour. I jumped at the chance, and my beautiful baby daughter, Jennifer Rose, was born on 24 February, a perfect, 7lb 2oz little girl.

Looking back, this should have been the happiest day of my life, but I have to admit now — and it hurts so deeply to think about it — her birth triggered off so many feelings that I suppose I suffered from shock. I was not mentally prepared for the birth of a live baby; I had not bought or sorted out one thing for the birth. Everything I had thought of doing I had convinced myself that I would be tempting fate. So when my baby arrived, fit and healthy (and hungry!), I was absolutely unprepared. The first night after I had her I woke up trembling with fear and shivering, and looking back now I know I was grieving for Christopher. I was so confused. Sometimes I thought I had given birth to him again and when Jennifer wanted feeding I couldn't relate to it, she seemed alien to me. I really couldn't understand what was happening to me. I loved her dearly and just yearned to feel normal.

I tried desperately hard to breastfeed Jennifer but the breastfeeding made me physically ill. I would sweat and shiver and I was actually sick. My husband got very worried about me and realised that something was very wrong. He had never seen me in such a state. I felt less able to cope with things than I had felt after the death of Christopher and my mum. I am usually a very strong, positive person, and I found myself unable to organise the simplest task. It was a big hurdle just to get dressed.

My husband talked to the midwife and mentioned that the way I felt seemed to be connected to the breastfeeding. So it was decided to drop the breastfeeding for twenty-four hours and see what happened. The change was incredible. Overnight I was almost back to my normal self and within a couple of days everything was all right. I suddenly felt all that I should have felt at the time of Jennifer's birth, and since that time my love and feelings towards my little girl have been enormous. It is frightening to love someone to that extent, but every day my love is greater. She is now 2½ years old and I cannot imagine life without her. We know just how special the gift of a life is and I enjoy every moment I spend with her. We never take her for granted and watch her sleeping at night and feel near to tears sometimes. It is hard to explain the deep feelings of love and fierce protection we feel.

Now, when I think back to that awful period in our lives, I

realise that it really did give us values. We know it is important to treasure every day and try to make the most out of what you have in life as it is so short and you never know what is round the corner. If we think about that time too much it gets disturbing, so we tend to try to put it to the back of our minds, but we will never forget our first little son, Christopher James.

I am now pregnant again, after seeing the same specialist. This time, instead of getting pregnant on the first course of treatment, I had to wait until the fourth try, but finally I got there. The desperation wasn't the same as we had already got Jennifer. So far, the pregnancy has been uneventful and the anxiety, although still there, is not quite as extreme as before. I think it's because I am running around after Jennifer so much that I don't have the same time to think about it. But at night, if the baby is inactive, it still keeps coming back to me. It's something that will never go away. I feel very frightened sometimes.

I am trying to look forward to a perfect Christmas with two healthy children. There is nothing more I could wish for than that, and if everything goes OK I would think myself so lucky in so many ways.

**Early in December, Ann was again induced and gave birth to a healthy baby boy whom she has called Jordan.**

## KEVIN

**Kevin and Melissa's baby, Lara, was born by emergency caesarean and lived for fifteen hours. The story of her birth is on page 16. Lara was Kevin and Melissa's second daughter. Her older sister, Kaly, was 2 years old when Lara was born. Melissa's womb ruptured during her labour and she had to have a hysterectomy.**

Seventeen months since our sweet little girl left us, her life was so brief, and it still seems so unreal. A day does not go by when I don't think of her, although not always with sadness or tears. As everyone who has suffered a tragedy knows 'life goes on', but I can remember learning to hate that expression at the time of Lara's death, because it seemed to me that life should stand still or allow us to go back and put everything right.

I believe the experience has affected our philosophy of life. At the time we were positive, approaching people to save them the embarrassment of approaching us. Some people were very good and have continued to be so. Others found it very difficult and still have not been able to talk to us openly. This we find sad as we would rather people said something than nothing at all. On the other hand, Lara was only seen by Melissa, my dad and myself, no one else from family or friends saw her. Therefore they cannot imagine her as a person. Some almost treat our loss like an early miscarriage. But we know (Melissa having suffered two miscarriages previously) that there is no comparison, although miscarriage brings its own emotional problems. We know Lara was a perfectly-formed baby girl and we so wish more people could have seen her, although at the time it did not seem the right thing to do. We did not push our parents or bring Kaly to the hospital to see Lara. We wish so much we had done this.

Kaly is so precious, but we try hard not to spoil her. It almost seems unfair that so much is expected of her as we and grandparents pour our love into one child. Some mornings I wake and hear Kaly talking to her imaginary friends and how I wish it was her sister she was talking to. We do not really know how they would have got on, but Kaly seems so ready now for a sister.

We should not forget that Kaly too has lost a sister. She was aware of the upset at the time, seeing her mummy and daddy cry, nanny and grandads unhappy, and we have brought her up with the knowledge of Lara's birth and death in simple terms. She even refers to Lara by name as her sister 'who died'. Children handle death so simply — maybe adults could learn from them.

We still go over what happened, what caused our little girl's death. The hospital invited us back to talk to them and go through Melissa's notes. The worst thing is knowing that if Melissa had had a caesarean by 3.30 p.m. that day we would have two little girls with us now, and would perhaps be planning a third. But since Kaly was born naturally, natural birth was the recommended route, and even Melissa's size did not convince the doctors to consider an earlier caesar. If we became bitter and tried to lay blame, where would that take us? It would not bring Lara back, and may detract from the time and love we give Kaly.

There have been different hurdles to overcome during the last seventeen months. First there was my return to work. I can remember thinking at the time I would never work again. My job is sales-orientated and targets seemed so unimportant. I wondered if I would ever get back to normal. Eventually you do get back in the swing and day-to-day problems start taking over again, but it is worth pausing sometimes and remembering what is important. It is the people we love so much, not material things.

The Christmas after Lara's death was very difficult. Should we celebrate the end of what had been such a sad and tragic year for us? Looking at Kaly there was only one answer, we had to be positive. Kaly would be 3 years old in December and it was a time for her. Some friends who had a daughter of their own kindly invited us away for Christmas and this was the perfect answer.

Then came the major hurdle, the anniversary of Lara's birth and death. We thought we should approach this as a normal day with no special plans. As we awoke on the morning of her birth, Melissa was crying and I knew I had to be with her and Kaly. I telephoned the office and explained that I needed to take a day's holiday to be with my wife. I am not sure that my boss fully understood but anyone who has been through a loss of someone dear would understand our feelings. We decided to go for a walk, with Kaly riding her bike. The sun was shining and birds singing; it was lovely, if only it wasn't so sad. At the time of her birth, we went to the hospital and visited the chapel and laid a yellow rosebud in memory of her. The following day we went to the crematorium and as I read our dedication in the memorial book, my tears began as if we had just lost our daughter.

What does the future hold? We are currently pursuing adoption but this is long and drawn out, with regular setbacks. We do not wish to replace Lara — all children are different and she must never be forgotten — but we do hope for a larger family. We have suffered a dual grief, the loss of a child and Melissa's hysterectomy. Our choice for more children has been taken from us. But we are blessed with a dear daughter, and have had the joy of a successful birth and the memories of the homecoming for the first time with a new baby. Many people do not experience this joy. On the other hand, many friends are phoning with news of their second or third pregnancies. We try to share their joy but deep down we can never feel the same about pregnancy. Also, for us the world seems full of couples with two children.

One of our strongest feelings now is to help others who have gone through a similar experience. Melissa is involved in talks and does voluntary work. It is so important to talk. To bottle it up only isolates you, and the experience, although so sad, doesn't have to make you a sadder person. We wish so much that this hadn't happened to us, but it has and we cannot change it. Life is for living and we must carry on in a positive way, for our own sakes and for the memory of Lara, who is always tucked away with us in the corner of our hearts.

## JOAN

**Joan lost her baby son when she was seventeen weeks pregnant. Her story is on page 18. The hospital where Joan was cared for did not at that time offer burial for babies born dead before twenty-eight weeks of pregnancy. But Joan knew that she needed to bury her baby, and insisted that she should be allowed to do so. The hospital has now changed its practice.**

Two years have passed since we lost our baby. The pain has ceased and the crying has eased. I still think of him every day, and some days I get very low. Looking back, I still feel very sad about having to fight to have a say in what happened to my baby's body, and I still get upset about having to leave hospital not knowing what was going to happen to him. Doctors and consultants can be so cold.

It gives me peace of mind to know where my baby's little body lies. Even though I don't visit his grave so often now, it is a sign he really did exist. I also have a photo of him. It all helps so much.

Eileen, the maternity unit administrator, has done a lot to change things at the hospital since our baby died, especially for early losses. It is now policy for all babies to be taken to the mortuary for three days, so that parents, upset at the time, still have a chance to see and hold their baby and are able to decide the future of their baby's body. The midwife also takes photos for parents to have if they wish. Attitudes are slowly changing, which can only be good for everyone, from parents right up to consultants. Staff are encouraged to go on counselling courses, and most are happy to do so.

I found after losing my baby that lots of friends did not know what to say to me. Some would try and pretend they hadn't seen me. In the end, I would put on a brave face and say hello very loudly. I think they were frightened I was going to burst into tears in the middle of the street and embarrass them. Of course, I felt like crying, but I talked about something else and broke the ice for them. Luckily I did have two friends I could talk to — it helped so much. They must have got fed up with me going over and over the same old things time and time again. I really appreciated it.

I found it practically impossible to find someone to talk to who had been through the same thing; it would have been nice to have that because of the strange things I thought and did. I thought I was going mad. I wore the same nightie that I'd worn the night I lost the baby for two weeks. It was covered in blood. Then, when I eventually washed it, I packed it away and never wore it again. I used to think of the baby waking up in the grave, being cold. This really upset me. I found a cuddly toy belonging to my daughter, Carla, and I would cuddle it, rocking in the chair. I also experienced severe mood swings from being really happy to getting really angry, throwing things around, hitting myself. I suppose looking back I blame myself for my baby dying.

Unfortunately for Carla, I still find it very hard to let her out of my sight when she is with me. Luckily for her, I go to work, so she does get a break. I think I realise now that life ends with a snap of the fingers. I explained to Carla why I am like this and hopefully she understands. It is getting better as she gets older.

My husband did not help much at the time. He thought that after one week I should be getting over it and back to normal. I don't think he really felt that. I think he just couldn't cope with me not being there for him.

About eighteen months after our baby died, my niece had a baby. I cried for days and could not bring myself to visit her, although we were quite close. It took nearly three months before I could hold the baby. I felt really guilty, but I couldn't help it.

As yet I have not been able to fall pregnant again. I have been having lots of tests which have all come back positive, although I have been told that they cannot guarantee that I will be able to carry a baby full term. But we are not giving up. We will leave it in God's hands.

## HAYRIYE

**Hayriye's second son, Serdar, died three months after he was born. He suffered brain damage and never came home from hospital. Hayriye's story is on page 20. She wrote this account sixteen months after Serdar's death.**

I can never hide my grief. I cry openly, even now. I am told it is wrong to cry. But it's more wrong to bottle it up inside. There are only a few people in the family that will talk to me about Serdar. My mum tells me not to go on and on about it. But I need to talk. Once I talk and cry and get it out I feel a bit better, until it builds up again and I need to let it out. I've had counselling since Serdar was born and right up to the present day. I became very depressed, very low. I made a big picture of Serdar, framed it and hung it on the wall opposite his brother's one. I looked at it and cried. People told me to take it down but I wouldn't. He's my son too — part of this family too — and loved the same. I had a longing to hold him again, I wanted to reach out and touch him. I knew he was gone, yet he was never really gone.

My doctor prescribed pills for me. She said it wasn't fair on my husband and other son that I can't get over it. She told me to be strong and tell myself I will get over it. Seven months later I went to see her again. I was in a terrible state. I didn't want to live. I wanted to go and be with Serdar. The doctor arranged for a psychiatrist to visit me at home. He prescribed a mild anti-depressant to lift my mood. I didn't like taking the pills as they made me drowsy and I had a toddler to run round after. A month ago I was referred to another psychiatrist. He told me I didn't need medication but I needed to talk. After I talk, I calm down. I told the doctor I feel as if I can't be happy again. I don't know how to be. He told me that that feeling of happiness isn't lost, it is still there but it's been buried underneath. There is a lot to clear out of the way before I can feel it again. This honestly makes sense to me.

My health visitor still visits me every few weeks. She got

Serhan, my older son, a place in the local nursery because the sadness was affecting him. The nursery is good for him and for me too. I help out there once a week and I enjoy it. I feel better now than I did a year ago, and another year on I'll feel better still.

You know, when the doctor spoke to us on the day Serdar died, she said it would have been better for me if Serdar had died at birth. I strongly disagree, but I do feel bitter that Serdar suffered that way. At least I had three months with him, we got to know and love him, and I have all my memories and photos. All those little things only I saw: the time he pulled my hair, made noises when I put him into the bath, carried on sucking even after he'd finished his milk, and smiled in his sleep. And he'd look deep into my eyes as I held and talked to him. Amongst all the sorrow, there were happy moments too. This time was better than none at all.

I know I'll never forget, I don't want to forget. But one day I'd like to be able to remember Serdar without being cut to pieces. Time makes it easier to live with, and accepting it is most of the battle. Letting go is not betrayal.

## VAL

**Val describes the birth of her twin girls, Samantha and Kathryn, on page 23. Samantha (Sammy) lived, but Kathryn died one day later.**

It is still very difficult for us on our surviving daughter's birthday. We feel great sadness that we aren't celebrating two birthdays. Last year Sammy was 3 years old and that was the worst birthday so far. Who says it gets easier? It seems to me it mustn't.

When Sammy was one, I thought, 'This must be the worst one to get over.' I just wanted to get the day over with, but at the same time of course it was Sammy's birthday. After all, she was one year old. I should be so happy that she had actually lived to be one. Up to her being one year old, I had the greatest fear that she was going to die, so when she was one year old I was relieved that she'd made it. But all I could think about was the fact that I should be celebrating Kathryn's birthday as well — two babies not one. We got the day over with. Sammy had a party and I tried my best to be happy for her. I said to her, and to Michael, my older son, 'Don't forget it's Kathryn's birthday today as well.'

The day after Sammy's first birthday was Kathryn's anniversary. We dreaded it months, weeks and days before it finally came. We tried to make it a short day. We went to bed really early to end the day quicker.

On Sammy's second birthday, and Kathryn's second anniversary, it wasn't so bad. We still dreaded it, but it wasn't as bad as the first and I thought, 'Mmm, time must be healing.'

When it came to Sammy's third birthday, we weren't looking forward to it, but we weren't dreading it as much. I had arranged that I would take cakes and so on to the mothers and toddlers group, and Sammy would have her party there. I was among lots of friends and just before we were due to sing 'Happy Birthday', it hit me. I ran into the kitchen and cried my heart out. Two friends put their arms round me and comforted me. They realised why I was crying. When I had stopped, we went in and sang 'Happy Birthday' and I couldn't sing for crying.

## SHARON

**A routine scan during Sharon's pregnancy showed that her daughter Sarah was anencephalic. Sharon and her partner, Ian, decided to terminate the pregnancy. Sharon's story is on page 26.**

During the months after the death of my daughter, we had to decide whether or not to go ahead and have another pregnancy. Before we made our decision, we went for genetic counselling. The doctors worked out that there was a one in 10 chance of it happening again. Would we risk it?

Well, a few months went by and we decided to have another baby. In September I was pregnant with our third child, and so the cycle begins again. Our baby was due in April. We went through the next few weeks wondering whether the baby was going to be all right. At fourteen weeks I had an early scan: 'The baby is fine,' the doctor said, 'but you have a cyst on your right ovary. I will have to make you an appointment to see your doctor.' I was so relieved to hear that the baby was fine, I never asked about the cyst.

I attended the doctor only to be told that the cyst would have to be removed. So at seventeen weeks pregnant I went back into the same ward where I lost Sarah a few months earlier, not knowing if I was going to lose this baby too. Thankfully the operation went well. I continued to carry my pregnancy and at thirty-eight and a half weeks I gave birth to a baby daughter, Rachel.

At first it was difficult to come to terms with having a baby girl, not only because I had lost a baby girl previously but also because I had a caesarean. I felt cheated of the birth and that I had made no real effort to deliver her.

The following February I had to have further surgery to remove the rest of my right ovary. Since then I miscarried at nine weeks. The doctor said the baby hadn't formed correctly. I sometimes wonder if it was another anencephalic and it was God's way of making us not have to make another decision as we had to make for Sarah.

I am so grateful for the support my husband and I have had throughout the past three years from doctors, nurses, friends and our mums and dads. I don't know how I would have got through without their love and support, and freedom to talk about our daughter. She is as much a part of our family as our other two children, even though we never got an opportunity to develop a relationship with her. We will never forget her and attend her grave often.

## PENNY

**Penny's son, Ryan, lived for four days. She had been told during her pregnancy that he would not survive, and he was expected to die before he was born. She tells about Ryan's birth and death on page 28.**

It's been over two years now since I lost Ryan. I have to keep counting the months to check because it still feels as if it all happened yesterday. The first year after he died is almost a complete blank. All I really remember is visits to the doctor, endless sleeping tablets and antidepressants. Unless people tell me what happened, it's all a blank — even Christmas and my twenty-first birthday.

I did manage to get a part-time job in the evenings but I had terrible panic attacks while I was there and I couldn't wait to get home. I also hated going out during the day. If I had somebody with me, I wasn't too bad, but if I had to go on my own, it was a real effort. I felt as if everyone was looking at me, that they knew I'd lost a baby and blamed me — even total stangers, I convinced myself that they were watching me. It got to the stage where I would only go out once a week, to the doctor's. Anything else was left to my husband to do after he finished work.

As the first anniversary of Ryan's death got closer, family and friends seemed to be telling me all the time to 'pull myself together'. I got really angry then. (Now I can see they were worried about me.) I used to think, 'How dare they tell me to pull myself together? They have no idea how I feel. How could they possibly understand?' I thought if I didn't cry every day people would think I'd 'got over' Ryan's death and I didn't want that. I loved him and missed him so much it hurt. If I didn't show it, how would people know?

About seven months after Ryan died, my husband started talking about us trying for another baby, and after days and days of talking, I reluctantly stopped taking the pill. Not that I ever needed it. Our sex-life was almost non-existent. I hated anything that made me think of babies. If I couldn't have Ryan, I didn't want any other.

The first anniversary came, and we cried and cried, but we coped. I didn't want to cope. I prayed that night to go to sleep and never wake up, but I did wake up, and life had to carry on. For days afterwards I felt terrible. I was walking around like a zombie until about two weeks after it hit me — I was pregnant again. I didn't need a test to confirm it, I just knew. My husband was overjoyed, I just felt sick. I wouldn't let him tell anyone, even our parents. I thought if I ignored it, it would go away. But it didn't of course, and when we did tell everyone, they were really happy for us. In fact, everyone was happy except me. I felt so guilty, as if I was betraying Ryan. I didn't want another baby, but at the same time I didn't want anything to happen to the baby I was carrying.

I had a scan at fifteen weeks and everything seemed fine, so I carried on as usual. I was beginning to get used to being pregnant again. I still felt guilty, but not as much. I realised I could love my daughter (who was 2), Ryan and my unborn baby all at the same time.

A week later I was rushed into hospital. I had started bleeding at work, which was how everything had started to go wrong with Ryan. I was told just to lie down and wait. I was convinced I was going to lose this baby, so I just switched off. I had another scan the next morning and everything was OK, but I took no notice. After a week of bed rest, I was allowed home. The bleeding had been 'just one of those things', nothing to worry about.

The following months went so slowly. I gave up work because I was so sure I would lose the baby. I began to hate my baby. I know that's a terrible thing to say but I was so convinced I would lose it that the longer I was pregnant the worse I became. At first, Wayne, my husband, said I was being silly, but towards the end of my pregnancy even he was worried by my attitude.

Finally, six days after my due date, I went into labour and half an hour after getting to the hospital, I gave birth to a beautiful, 6lb 7oz baby girl. When the nurse gave her to me, I took one look at her and forgot I was supposed to hate her. She was perfect in every way. As I looked into her eyes, for a split second I was holding Ryan again. They were so alike. It was as if Ryan was letting me know it was OK to love her.

If someone had told me two years ago that I could be this happy, I would never have believed it. Looking back from today, I like to think I'm one of the lucky ones. I still love and miss Ryan, and cry myself to sleep some nights. But when I think what I have got, I'm satisfied — two beautiful, healthy daughters and a wonderful, precious memory that no one can ever hurt, or change, or take away from me.

# APPENDIX 1
# Medical Explanations

In the UK at present, 5 babies in every thousand are stillborn, and 5 more die within the first four weeks of life. So, 10 in every thousand babies, or one in every hundred, are stillborn or die shortly after birth. This figure does not include babies who are born dead or miscarry before twenty-eight weeks gestation, as these babies are not registered and do not enter the statistics.

Every time a baby dies perhaps the most urgent immediate question is why? What could have caused the death? Could it have been prevented? Sometimes a clear cause is found, but often parents find that there is no satisfactory medical explanation, because there is still so much that is not understood about pregnancy and about the different things that can affect the development of a baby. At the present time, no clear cause can be found even after a detailed post-mortem for about half of all stillbirths. And even when it is possible to say why a baby died during pregnancy or labour, it is often not possible to explain what started the chain of events that led to that death. In the case of a premature baby who has died after birth, the final cause of death is more often understood. But although doctors understand why some premature babies die, they still do not always understand why some labours begin too early. So, for a large number of parents, a full explanation of their baby's death is simply not possible at present and may never be.

But all parents want and need to understand why, in medical terms, their baby died, or at least they want to know as much as it is possible to know. We hope that this chapter will confirm and clarify for many parents what they have already been told by the professionals caring for them and their baby. Other parents may wish to go back to their doctors or other professionals to ask further questions. We hope that this chapter will help them to do this.

## Medical knowledge and professional judgement

We have outlined what is known about why babies die before or shortly after birth under the headings listed below. In some cases the explanations are quite clear. In others they may seem frustratingly unclear. This is because, despite extensive and continuing research, there is still much that is not understood or is uncertain about how a baby develops in the womb and what affects this process.

In these areas of uncertainty, doctors and midwives often have to rely on their own professional judgement and experience when caring for pregnant women and their babies. For this reason, there can be major differences between the approach of one consultant and another, even within the same hospital. There may also be differences in hospital practice because of variations in resources. Some hospitals are equipped with the latest high-tech equipment for diagnosis and treatment; others are not. We have tried to give the current views and practices of the majority of obstetricians and paediatricians, but there will be some professionals who disagree, both with our understanding of the problem, and with our description of the treatments and preventive measures that may be used.

Doctors and midwives sometimes find it very difficult to say when they are uncertain or simply do not know why something is going or has gone wrong, especially in the highly-charged situations of pregnancy, labour and neonatal care. Very often they feel they should know.

For parents too, until they have experienced the loss of a baby, it can seem that medicine and science now have an answer to all obstetric problems and can control pregnancy and its outcome. More is heard about the successes of obstetric and neonatal medicine than about the failures and continuing uncertainties. Many tests can now be carried out during pregnancy to detect problems, but parents may not have realised that often, once a problem has been detected, little or nothing can be done to put it right. The message often put across in antenatal clinics is that if parents are obedient and careful they will be rewarded with a perfectly healthy baby. All parents naturally want and expect certainty, knowledge and a successful outcome, and it may be difficult to accept doubt and uncertainty in the professionals they encounter. But for bereaved parents, part of understanding the cause of their baby's death, may be understanding what is not known or what is uncertain or contentious.

## Medical language

In this chapter, we have included some of the technical terms doctors and other professionals commonly use for their own convenience and for precision when discussing symptoms, causes and conditions. People who are not familiar with these terms can easily be put off and may even come to feel, wrongly, that they are not capable of understanding what is going on. This makes it difficult for parents to believe that they are the key participants in the situation, and that they are entitled to ask questions and to clarify confusions.

However, in most cases there is nothing particularly mysterious or difficult about what is being described in medical terms. Medical language is just a set of alternative words describing ideas which we are usually familiar with and can understand quite well. For example, *pyrexia* simply means a raised temperature, *pulmonary* means to do with the lungs, *hypoplasia* means underdeveloped and *haemorrhage* means bleeding. In most cases it is not difficult for professionals to translate their message into plain English and to fill in any gaps in our understanding of the human body, but often doctors and others are no longer aware of what is and is not easy for a non-medical person to understand.

Parents have every right to ask for an explanation in language they can understand. We hope that the medical terms we have used in this chapter will help increase their confidence and encourage them to ask — and to keep on asking — as many questions as they wish until they feel they understand.

## The problems of simplification

The human body consists of an extraordinarily complicated combination of systems which all affect and are affected by each other. In trying to outline different causes and effects, we have focused on what we understand to be the most important and direct chains of events and have left out many things that are going on at the same time. This has enabled us to be fairly brief and, we hope, clear. At the same time, it has inevitably involved judgements about what is and is not significant, and has meant omitting a lot of detail. Readers who would like to find out more about a particular subject may like to speak to their own GP or consultant, or to look at some of the books listed on page 243.

They may also like to contact one of the many voluntary groups offering information, advice and support for parents whose baby has died and/or who are considering another pregnancy after a bereavement. Some of these (for example, the Miscarriage Association, the Stillbirth and Neonatal Death Society [SANDS] and the Nippers Bereavement Support Group) exist to provide general support for parents whose baby has died. Others (such as the Sickle Cell Society and the Association for Spina Bifida and Hydrocephalus [ASBAH]) provide support and information about specific conditions. Relevant voluntary organisations in the UK are referred to in the text and are listed on pages 245–50.

## MEDICAL EXPLANATIONS: CONTENTS LIST

### PROBLEMS IN PREGNANCY AND AFFECTING THE BABY'S DEVELOPMENT

**Infections in the mother** (page 190)

> organisms that can cross the placenta; cytomegalovirus, human parvovirus B19, listeriosis, rubella (German measles), toxoplasmosis (page 190)
> organisms that can cause premature labour; urinary tract infections (page 193)

**Other problems to do with the mother's health** (page 194)

> diabetes (page 195)
> epilepsy (page 197)
> high blood pressure (page 197)
> kidney disease (page 198)
> sickle cell disease (page 199)
> systemic lupus erythematosus (lupus) (page 200)

**Problems to do with the baby's development** (page 201)

> chromosome abnormalities; Edwards' syndrome, Patau's syndrome (page 202)
> neural tube defects; anencephaly, spina bifida (page 205)
> hydrocephalus (hydrocephaly) (page 207)
> rhesus disease; hydrops fetalis (page 209)
> congenital heart problems; hypoplastic left-heart syndrome, transposition of the great vessels, other congenital heart defects (page 211)
> other congenital problems; Potter's syndrome (page 215)
> twins and other multiple pregnancies (page 217)
> alpha thalassaemia major (page 218)

*PROBLEMS DURING LABOUR*

**Problems to do with the placenta** (page 220)

> placental abruption (abruptio placentae) (page 220)
> placental failure (page 220)

**Problems to do with the umbilical cord** (page 220)

> prolapsed cord (page 221)

true knot (page 221)
cord around the neck (page 221)

**Birth asphyxia** (page 222)

fetal distress (page 222)
meconium aspiration (page 223)
babies who do not breathe (page 224)

## PROBLEMS AFTER BIRTH

**Premature babies** (page 224)

causes of premature labour (page 225)
complications for premature babies (page 226)

**Problems to do with the baby's lungs** (page 227)

respiratory distress syndrome (page 228)
pneumonia (page 228)
persistent pulmonary hypertension/persistent fetal circulation
(page 229)
bronchopulmonary dysplasia (page 229)

**Intraventricular haemorrhage** (page 230)

**Infections** (page 230)

organisms that can affect babies at the time of delivery; group
B streptococcus, herpes, chicken pox (page 231)
secondary infections; meningitis, pneumonia, septicaemia
(blood poisoning) (page 233)

**Necrotising enterocolitis** (page 234)

# PROBLEMS IN PREGNANCY AND AFFECTING THE BABY'S DEVELOPMENT

## PROBLEMS TO DO WITH THE PLACENTA

The placenta, also called the afterbirth, connects the baby to the mother's body. It grows with the baby and is implanted in the lining of the mother's womb. The placenta acts as the baby's lungs, kidneys and bowel while the baby is in the womb. It allows oxygen, nutrients and antibodies (which protect the baby from certain infections) to pass from the mother to the baby, and the baby's waste products to pass back to the mother for disposal. The placenta also produces hormones which are needed to maintain the pregnancy.

The baby has its own separate blood circulation system. Blood passes round the baby's body, along the umbilical cord to the placenta, and back again to the baby's body. The baby's circulation system is quite separate from the mother's. This is essential to ensure that the mother's immune system does not reject the baby in the same way as a kidney patient's immune system sometimes rejects a transplanted kidney. Although the mother's and the baby's circulation systems are quite separate, they run very closely alongside each other in the placenta, so that the baby's blood vessels are surrounded in the placenta by the mother's blood. This enables essential oxygen, nutrients and waste products to pass between the two circulation systems through the very thin walls of the blood vessels.

The placenta is vital to the baby throughout pregnancy and during labour, up to the time when the baby is delivered and can begin to breathe for itself. Once the baby is born, the placenta comes away from the wall of the womb, and is delivered through the vagina.

PLACENTAL INSUFFICIENCY AND PLACENTAL FAILURE
Placental insufficiency is sometimes called placental dysfunction. It occurs when the placenta is not working efficiently, has not developed properly, or does not keep growing with the baby. Placental insufficiency can also happen if the mother's circulatory system is not working properly because of high blood pressure or other chronic disease. As a result, the baby does not get enough oxygen or nourishment, becomes weak and does not grow properly.

In severe cases the placenta is unable to provide the baby with enough oxygen and the baby dies in the womb. This is often known as placental failure. Placental failure is most likely to occur from twenty-eight weeks gestation onwards when the baby's growth usually accelerates rapidly. There may be little or no warning, and there may be no history of placental insufficiency. The baby may simply slow down and then stop moving. (See also Placental failure, page 220.)

The causes of placental insufficiency and placental failure are not yet fully understood. Known causes include maternal blood pressure that remains high for some time (see High blood pressure, page 197, and Pregnancy-induced hypertension, page 188) and infections or blockages (infarctions) which affect the mother's blood supply to the placenta.

It is not always possible to diagnose placental insufficiency but it may be suspected if the baby becomes less active or is not growing as expected (also known as small for dates or intra-uterine growth retardation — that is, delayed growth within the womb). If placental insufficiency is suspected, the baby's growth may be checked regularly by ultrasound scan. Wherever possible, the causes of placental insufficiency are treated so that the baby's growth improves, but often there is little or nothing that can be done to help the baby grow, even after placental insufficiency is confirmed.

Babies who are born small for dates are at increased risk of infection and other problems such as low sugar or calcium levels. These risks increase further if a baby is also premature.

**Incidence:** Placental insufficiency and placental failure linked with pregnancy-induced hypertension (see page 188) are most common in first pregnancies. They are less likely to recur in further pregnancies with the same partner.

**Another pregnancy:** If placental insufficiency is suspected doctors will usually carry out regular ultrasound scans to check the baby's growth rate. They may also carry out other checks on the baby's health such as heart rate traces or Doppler blood flow studies, which use reflected sound waves to examine the blood flow through the umbilical cord and the placenta and check how much oxygen is getting through. However, as mentioned above, it is not always possible to do anything to increase a baby's rate of growth.

## PLACENTAL DEGENERATION

The placenta usually reaches its peak of efficiency near the end of pregnancy. In some cases it begins to deteriorate too early or too fast causing placental insufficiency or placental failure (see above). Usually no cause can be found for placental degeneration but it can follow pregnancy-induced hypertension (see page 188), chronic high blood-pressure (see page 197), or other problems in the mother.

## ANTEPARTUM HAEMORRHAGE

Any bleeding during pregnancy after twenty-eight weeks gestation may be called an antepartum haemorrhage (that is, bleeding before delivery). Antepartum haemorrhage occurs in about 3 per cent of all pregnancies. The two main causes are placental abruption and placenta praevia which are described below.

## PLACENTAL ABRUPTION (ABRUPTIO PLACENTAE)

Occasionally, bleeding between the placenta and the wall of the womb to which it is attached causes the placenta to become partly or wholly separated (abrupted) from the wall of the womb. This reduces or cuts off the supply of oxygen and nutrients to the baby. Placental abruption can happen at any time during pregnancy but is most usual towards the end.

Sometimes the placenta only separates slightly from the womb. The mother may have some visible vaginal bleeding and possibly some pain but with rest and luck, the pregnancy continues. However, even slight placental abruption may cause premature labour, and the baby may be born too young to survive.

In severe placental abruption, all or most of the placenta separates from the womb, and the baby's oxygen supply is cut off. Sometimes the bleeding is contained within the womb and is not visible. Severe placental abruption is usually very painful for the mother. In an emergency, doctors perform a caesarean section as soon as possible to try to save both mother and baby. The mother may need an urgent blood transfusion to replace the blood she loses, especially since, in a severe case of placental abruption, her blood may not clot.

In some cases the baby dies because of lack of oxygen following

MEDICAL EXPLANATIONS · 183

the separation of the placenta from the womb. If the baby is born alive, lack of oxygen can sometimes cause severe brain damage, and also, if there has been a major loss of blood, anaemia. In babies born very prematurely after placental abruption, there is an increased risk of respiratory distress syndrome (see page 228).

No clear cause can be found for about half the cases of placental abruption. It is sometimes associated with pregnancy-induced hypertension (see page 188), but nobody understands what causes that either. It is also more common among heavy smokers. In extremely rare cases, placental abruption can be caused by a serious injury to the mother's stomach after a fall or other accident.

**Another pregnancy:** Placental abruption is very unlikely to recur in another pregnancy. However, women who have lost a baby from abruption may be offered induction about two weeks before their due date in another pregnancy. This can reduce both parents' and obstetricians' anxieties.

PLACENTA PRAEVIA

The placenta is normally implanted in the upper part of the mother's womb (called the fundus). Placenta praevia is the term used when the placenta lies very low in the womb, partly or wholly blocking the entrance to the birth canal. When the lower part of the womb stretches in late pregnancy, a low-lying placenta may separate from the wall of the womb and bleeding may occur. If the mother goes into labour, the placenta may separate further from the womb as the cervix opens, causing severe and dangerous maternal bleeding and cutting off the baby's blood supply. The baby must be delivered urgently by caesarean section. If the baby has been deprived of oxygen, he or she may die or be severely brain damaged.

**Another pregnancy:** Placenta praevia may be diagnosed by ultrasound scan at sixteen to eighteen weeks. However, many placentas seem low at this stage, and the situation is normally reviewed at about thirty-two weeks. If placenta praevia is confirmed at this stage, doctors will plan to deliver the baby by caesarean section, usually at thirty-seven weeks unless bleeding occurs earlier.

HYDATIDIFORM MOLE

Very occasionally an error occurs when the chromosomes are forming in an egg (see Chromosome abnormalities page 202) causing a hydatidiform mole. This is a condition of the placenta in which the fertilised egg does not develop properly and no baby develops. The placenta grows very fast, forming thousands of small fluid-filled cysts the size of grapes. Although there is no baby, the placenta usually causes the womb to expand abnormally fast. The rapid growth of the placenta raises the woman's hormone level so she may have severe nausea, vomiting and even high blood pressure. She may also have vaginal bleeding. A hydatidiform mole is also called a molar pregnancy.

In most cases, a hydatidiform mole is expelled spontaneously. If not, it is normally diagnosed by ultrasound scan and by a raised level of the hormone human chorionic gonadotrophin (HCG). The apparent pregnancy is usually terminated immediately and the womb carefully emptied to ensure that no tissue from the mole remains.

Very rarely, a hydatidiform mole may become cancerous. This cancer, called choriocarcinoma, is almost always curable if it is caught in time. After a hydatidiform mole, a woman will have frequent tests to make sure that a cancer is not developing. Provided the test results are normal for six months or a year, the woman is usually advised that she can try for another baby.

**Incidence:** Hydatidiform moles occur in about one in 2,000 pregnancies in the UK. A woman who has already had a hydatidiform mole has a one in 50 risk of having another. There is a slight tendency for hydatidiform moles to run in families, and they are slightly more common in women of South-East Asian origin.

## PROBLEMS TO DO WITH THE WOMB

Abnormalities and problems to do with the womb can cause premature labour, especially in the middle months of pregnancy. As a result, babies may be born too young to survive. With improved neonatal intensive care, it is increasingly possible to treat and save babies who are delivered very early. Even so, babies born before thirty weeks are still very much at risk (see page 224).

**Another pregnancy:** In some cases a problem with the womb cannot be completely cured, so parents who are considering another pregnancy will need a good deal of practical and emotional support. If it seems possible that another baby might be born very prematurely, the GP will usually refer parents during pregnancy to a hospital with a very skilled neonatal intensive care unit, where babies as young as twenty-three weeks can sometimes survive.

## WEAK CERVIX (INCOMPETENT CERVIX)

The cervix is a tight ring of muscle between the vagina and the womb. It normally remains closed during pregnancy until the baby is ready to be delivered. During labour, it opens wide to let the baby out of the womb. Very occasionally, a woman has a weak cervix (doctors often use the term incompetent cervix) which opens up and causes the baby to be delivered too early. This usually happens between the sixteenth and twenty-fourth week of pregnancy, when the baby is still too young to survive.

There are several causes of a weak cervix. Very rarely, a woman is born with one. More often, it seems to be the result of surgery or other past events, for example, a D and C (dilation and curettage) to empty the womb after an earlier miscarriage, a difficult forceps delivery, the rapid delivery of a very large baby, a cone biopsy to remove cancerous cells in the cervix or a previous late termination of pregnancy. Doctors are now very aware of the consequences of damaging the cervix and take great care to be as gentle as possible during all these procedures. If a woman is carrying twins or more babies, the additional pressure on her cervix, whether it is weak or not, may cause it to open up, leading to premature labour.

The first sign of a cervix opening is usually the waters breaking without warning in the middle of the pregnancy. There may also be some bleeding. The mother then usually has a short and often relatively painless labour. Unfortunately, a weak cervix is not usually diagnosed until after a baby has already been lost, and even then it can be difficult to be sure of the diagnosis. There is at present no reliable diagnostic test for a weak cervix.

**Incidence:** There is a good deal of debate among obstetricians about how often the loss of a baby in the middle of pregnancy is genuinely due to a weak cervix and how often it has some other cause. As a result, estimates of the incidence of a weak cervix in the UK vary from one in 100 to one in 2,000.

**Another pregnancy:** Doctors may suggest inserting a stitch (cerclage) at the upper end of the cervix to try to hold the cervix closed until the baby is ready to be born. There are several slightly different types of stitch, named after the obstetricians who invented them. The main ones are Macdonald and Shirodkar. A cervical stitch is inserted under a general anaesthetic, usually at about fourteen to sixteen weeks of pregnancy. This is after the time when most miscarriages due to chromosomal abnormalities would have occurred. The stitch is put through the cervix and pulled tight, rather like a drawstring on a shoe bag. Provided labour has not begun earlier, the stitch is removed during the thirty-eighth week of the pregnancy.

There is much debate about the effectiveness of a cervical stitch in maintaining a pregnancy in a woman who has a weak cervix. Some doctors feel that bed rest may have an equally important role to play. However, interim results from a major randomised controlled trial (which is still continuing) show that a cervical stitch can help prevent some premature labours in cases of 'true cervical incompetence'. But the cervical stitch also has disadvantages. One is the increased possibility of infection due to the presence of a foreign body in the system. Another is that following the stitch there is usually more medical intervention throughout the pregnancy, with more frequent stays in hospital during pregnancy, and higher rates of induced labour and caesarean section. Although many women with a weak cervix feel that a cervical stitch offers their only hope of maintaining a pregnancy, the decision should always be well informed.

For support and contact with women who have had a cervical stitch, contact the Cervical Stitch Network, see page 246 for address.

FIBROIDS

A fibroid is a non-cancerous growth in the wall of the womb. During pregnancy, the high levels of the hormone oestrogen can cause the fibroid to grow rapidly. Occasionally fibroids can distort the inside of the womb so that the mother goes into premature labour. If the fibroids outgrow their blood supply they may also degenerate and cause pain.

**Incidence:** Fibroids tend to become more common as women get older, and are more common in women of African and West Indian origin.

**Another pregnancy:** If fibroids are found to be distorting the womb and are thought to have caused the previous premature labour, doctors may decide to operate to remove them when the woman is no longer pregnant. This is done under general anaesthetic and leaves a scar in the uterus where the fibroid has been removed. In a later pregnancy, the woman will be watched carefully, in the same way as someone who has a scar from a caesarean section, as there is thought to be a very slight danger that the scar may weaken. (See also Spontaneous premature labour, page 225.)

ABNORMALLY SHAPED WOMB
The womb is originally formed by two separate tubes which fuse together. Very rarely the fusion is not complete and a woman may be born with an abnormally shaped womb, divided to a greater or lesser extent by a wall of muscle down the middle. Some variations in the shape of the womb do not cause problems, but others do. If a woman has a womb that is completely or almost completely divided in half (forming a double womb), there may not be enough room for the baby as it grows. The mother may then go into premature labour before the baby is old enough to survive. Problems can also occur if the placenta implants itself onto a part of the womb that has a poor blood supply, causing placental insufficiency (see page 180).

An abnormally shaped womb is most likely to cause the loss of a baby in the middle period (fourth to sixth month) of a pregnancy. It is not possible to predict before pregnancy whether there are likely to be problems.

**Another pregnancy:** If an abnormal womb is suspected, it can be checked by a special X-ray called an HSG (hystero-salpingogram). This involves injecting a dye into the womb through the vagina to show the shape of the womb on the X-ray.

If a severely abnormal or double womb is found, some doctors may advise an operation when the woman is not pregnant. However, this is not always successful. It may leave a large scar which could prevent the implantation of fertilised eggs in future pregnancies and cause miscarriages. If a pregnancy succeeds, the woman will be watched carefully, in the same way as someone who has a scar from a caesarean section, as there is thought to be a very slight danger that the scar may weaken. If no operation is carried out, it is possible that in a future pregnancy the womb will stretch further and will retain the baby until he or she is old enough to survive birth.

Decisions about what to do about an abnormal womb can be very difficult and it is important that parents get the advice and support they need to make the decision that is right for them.´

## PROBLEMS IN THE MOTHER CAUSED BY PREGNANCY

### PREGNANCY-INDUCED HYPERTENSION (PIH)

Hypertension is the medical term for high blood pressure. Pregnancy-induced hypertension (that is, high blood pressure caused by pregnancy) is also known as hypertensive disease of pregnancy, and used to be called pre-eclampsia or pre-eclampsic toxaemia (PET). These changes in terminology indicate recent changes in medical understanding of the problem. However, the causes of pregnancy-induced hypertension are still not understood and there are widely differing views about the best way to manage it.

Pregnancy-induced hypertension is most likely to develop in the second half of pregnancy. The key symptom is raised blood pressure (hypertension) though it is not known what causes this. Another symptom is a raised level of protein in the mother's urine (proteinuria), and this can indicate an increased risk to the baby. Most women also have swelling (oedema) of the feet and hands and experience an increase in their weight due to water retention.

High blood pressure in pregnancy can cut down the exchange of oxygen, nutrients and waste products through the placenta, causing placental insufficiency (see page 180) and affecting the baby's growth. There is a high risk that pregnancy-induced hypertension will threaten the lives of both mother and baby if it is severe and prolonged or if it progresses to eclampsia (see below). Pregnancy-induced hypertension is more dangerous to the baby the earlier in pregnancy it begins.

If a mother develops severe pregnancy-induced hypertension or eclampsia (see below), the baby must be delivered immediately because both the mother's and the baby's lives are in danger as long as the pregnancy continues. The baby is at serious risk in the womb if the placenta has already been severely affected or has separated from the wall of the womb (see Placental abruption, page 182). In some cases, the baby has to be delivered very prematurely and may be too young to survive outside the womb.

Pregnancy-induced hypertension always disappears after delivery and the mother's blood pressure returns to normal unless she already had undetected hypertension (see High blood pressure, page 197) before she became pregnant.

**Incidence:** Pregnancy-induced hypertension is most likely to occur in first pregnancies and in subsequent pregnancies with a new partner. It occurs in about one in 8 of first pregnancies and in about one in 20 of all pregnancies. It seems to be more likely in all pregnancies where the mother has high blood pressure or kidney (renal) disease (see pages 197 and 198) before she becomes pregnant, if she is over 35, or if she is carrying two or more babies.

**Another pregnancy:** There is a good deal of debate about the prevention and management of pregnancy-induced hypertension, and little clear evidence of what helps. However, it now seems clear that, contrary to the advice that used to be given, women who are at risk of pregnancy-induced hypertension should not restrict the amount of salt they eat during pregnancy, nor try to restrict their weight gain. Some experts think that a high protein diet may help. It is unlikely that this will do any harm as part of an overall balanced diet.

For support and contact with other women who have had pregnancy-induced hypertension, contact the Pre-Eclamptic Toxaemia Society, see page 247 for address.

ECLAMPSIA

Eclampsia is a dangerous condition in which a mother develops very high blood pressure. She may see flashing lights in front of her eyes, have a severe headache and fits (due to the effect of the high blood pressure on her brain), a sharp pain in her stomach, and may lose consciousness. The mother's high blood pressure damages the placenta and can cause placental abruption (see page

182) and premature labour. The baby may die due to lack of oxygen unless delivered immediately, usually by emergency caesarean section. Eclampsia is also dangerous for the mother since very high blood pressure can damage her brain and other vital organs, such as the kidneys and the liver. It is treated as a medical emergency. The mother receives intensive drug and nursing care.

**Incidence:** Eclampsia is usually, but not always, preceded by pregnancy–induced hypertension (see above). It occurs in about one in every 1,000 deliveries in the UK. Eclampsia is most common in first pregnancies but occasionally recurs in future pregnancies. It usually occurs towards the end of pregnancy but can happen earlier or, occasionally, after delivery. It is more common if there are twins or more babies.

For support and contact with other women who have had eclampsia, contact the Pre-Eclamptic Toxaemia Society, see page 247.

## INFECTIONS IN THE MOTHER

Certain infections in the mother can be very dangerous to her developing baby. Some can cross the placenta and may cause the death of the baby in the womb. Others may cause the mother to go into premature labour and the baby may be born too young or too severely handicapped to live.

Most of these dangerous infections are rare and little is known about their precise effects or how many deaths they cause. This is partly because there is no accurate way of testing for many of these diseases during pregnancy. Sometimes, even if a test can be done, it is difficult to tell whether any antibodies found are due to a current active infection (which might harm the baby) or to a previous infection earlier in the woman's life (which will not). In addition, if an active infection is found there is usually no way of telling whether or how severely the baby might be affected, and there may be no effective treatment available.

The main infections that are known to have caused late miscarriages, stillbirths and neonatal deaths are outlined here.

ORGANISMS THAT CAN CROSS THE PLACENTA
The placenta prevents many organisms passing from the mother's

bloodstream to the baby. However, some organisms can cross the placenta and may damage the baby, especially in the first three months when the baby's organs are forming. In most cases, an affected baby miscarries early, but the following organisms are known occasionally to cause late miscarriage, stillbirth, handicap, or severe postnatal infection:

## Cytomegalovirus (CMV)

CMV is a virus transmitted by human contact, and is common in both children and adults. It usually causes only mild symptoms or passes unnoticed. But if a woman catches CMV during pregnancy, it may infect her baby in the womb. In most cases there are no lasting effects on the baby, but occasionally an overwhelming infection can cause stillbirth, death soon after birth or severe handicap. If a CMV infection is diagnosed during pregnancy it cannot be treated since there are at present no known suitable antiviral agents. There is also no vaccine against CMV.

**Another pregnancy:** CMV is most dangerous and most likely to infect a baby in the womb if the mother catches it for the first time during the pregnancy. The disease can recur but it is thought to be less likely to cross the placenta in future pregnancies.

For support and advice about cytomegalovirus, contact the Cytomegalovirus Support Group, see page 246.

## Human parvovirus B19

Human parvovirus is a common infection, especially in children, and is transmitted through human contact. It usually causes no symptoms, though people may feel slightly unwell and sometimes develop a rash. But if a woman catches human parvovirus during pregnancy, especially during the middle months, it can occasionally cross the placenta and infect the baby, sometimes causing miscarriage or stillbirth.

There are no figures available for the incidence of human parvovirus in the UK, nor for the number of babies who die as a result of their mother contracting the virus, but it is thought that the numbers are very small. There is at present no treatment or vaccination for human parvovirus.

## Listeriosis

Listeria is a bacteria which exists widely in the environment, for example in soil and vegetation, as well as in food. At any time, listeria is carried without symptoms by about one in 20 of the

UK population. Listeriosis (the disease) is most commonly contracted from food.

If a woman has listeriosis during pregnancy she may have no symptoms at all, she may develop a mild flu-like illness or she may be severely ill with symptoms similar to acute food poisoning and a high temperature. It is thought that the listeria bacteria can reach a baby by several different routes. It can pass into the womb either across the placenta or through the vagina (even if the membranes are intact), it can be caught in the birth canal during delivery or it can be caught from an infected person after delivery.

A baby who is severely affected in the womb may miscarry or be stillborn. A baby who is born with listeriosis or who catches it during delivery or soon after birth, may develop serious and often fatal infections such as pneumonia, septicaemia and meningitis (see pages 228 and 233). If the mother develops a very high temperature in pregnancy due to listeria, this by itself can start off labour and the baby may be born too young to live.

**Incidence:** The incidence of miscarriage, stillbirth and neonatal death due to listeriosis in the UK is low, but it is rising, probably due to increasing consumption of ready-cooked meals and soft cheeses.

**Another pregnancy:** It is thought that once a woman has had listeria she has some immunity and that even if she is infected again in a future pregnancy, this will probably not seriously affect the baby.

See page 130 for those foods that are most likely to carry the bacteria and for information about other ways of reducing the risk of listeriosis in pregnancy.

## Rubella

Rubella (German measles) is usually a mild disease in children and adults, sometimes causing a rash and a slight temperature. However, if it is caught in the first four months of pregnancy, and especially in the first ten weeks, it can cause severe developmental abnormalities in the baby, leading to miscarriage, stillbirth or severe handicap. It is caught through contact with an infected person. A person with rubella is infectious for about two weeks or a little longer, starting from five to seven days before the rash begins.

**Another pregnancy**: Once a person has had rubella they are almost always immune. Tests to check for immunity to rubella are available from GPs and family planning clinics as well as at antenatal clinics. Women who are not immune can be vaccinated when they are not pregnant. It is important not to conceive for three months after having the vaccination, and to have another blood test before conceiving, to check that the vaccination was successful. Some doctors advise all pregnant women to try and avoid contact with rubella whether or not they are immune.

For information and advice about rubella, contact SENSE (The National Deaf–Blind and Rubella Organisation), see page 247.

## Toxoplasmosis

This organism — toxoplasma gondii — usually produces mild symptoms or no symptoms at all in the mother but can infect a baby in the womb and cause serious problems, including hydrocephalus (see page 207), miscarriage, stillbirth, neonatal death and premature labour. Toxoplasmosis is usually caught from handling or eating raw or undercooked meat, or from touching the litter and faeces of infected cats.

The incidence of toxoplasmosis infection in the UK is unknown but is thought to be very low. During pregnancy, toxoplasmosis seems to be most dangerous to the baby during the first three months of gestation, though the likelihood of the virus crossing the placenta is smallest at this time.

**Another pregnancy**: It is thought that once a woman has had toxoplasmosis she develops some immunity which will protect future pregnancies. Tests for immunity to toxoplasmosis are available from GPs and antenatal clinics. See page 131 for information about avoiding sources of toxoplasmosis.

For contact and advice from people who have had toxoplasmosis, contact the Toxoplasmosis Trust, see page 247.

ORGANISMS THAT CAN CAUSE PREMATURE LABOUR
Certain organisms, including Group B streptococcus (see page 231), listeria (see above), mycoplasma and ureaplasma are known sometimes to cause premature labour. The mechanism is not always understood. It is thought that some bacteria, for example, listeria, affect the membranes that line the mother's womb. These membranes contain a substance similar to prostaglandin, a natural hor-

mone which stimulates labour and causes the membranes to rupture. Bacterial infection in the membranes may release this substance.

If a mother develops a high temperature from any cause during any stage of pregnancy, her womb may start to contract and her baby may be born prematurely. Severe kidney and chest infections are particularly dangerous as a cause of high temperatures leading to premature labour. For more about the complications of prematurity, see page 226.

## Urinary tract infections

The urinary tract consists of the kidneys, the ureters (through which urine flows from the kidneys to the bladder), the bladder and the urethra (through which urine is passed out of the body). During pregnancy, hormones cause the smooth muscles of the body to relax. The ureters become more open and bacterial infections can more easily travel up them to the kidneys.

In the UK, roughly one in every 100 women develops an inflammation of the bladder (cystitis) and/or an inflammation of the kidneys (pyelonephritis) during pregnancy. In the early stages there may be no signs, and the condition may flare up suddenly. Doctors will try to bring the infection under control with antibiotics, and to bring down the temperature by using drugs such as aspirin and paracetamol. If the mother's temperature remains very high the baby may be born prematurely.

**Another pregnancy**: A woman who has had a serious urinary tract infection in a previous pregnancy does not face any increased risk in future pregnancies unless she has an abnormal urinary tract or a chronic kidney problem which makes her more vulnerable to infection. In this case, her condition would be very carefully monitored throughout pregnancy. Should a problem arise, any symptoms or signs would be treated early.

## OTHER PROBLEMS TO DO WITH THE MOTHER'S HEALTH

Certain pre-existing medical conditions in a mother can increase the risks to her baby. In most cases, parents will have been able to discuss these conditions with doctors and others throughout the pregnancy, and will understand them fully.

**Another pregnancy**: In some cases, for example diabetes and epilepsy, the chances of a live healthy baby in a future pregnancy can be greatly increased with specialist pre-conceptual care, and parents who have not had this previously may wish to seek it out before they consider becoming pregnant again. If another baby is likely to be at risk, parents may also wish to be referred to a hospital with a very good neonatal intensive care unit for their antenatal care and/or for the delivery.

It is extremely important that parents have confidence in the professionals who are caring for them during another pregnancy, and that they are able to discuss their questions and worries fully. Some may choose to be referred to a specialist who has particular expertise in providing care for people with their particular condition.

For the National Childbirth Trust Contact Register for parents with particular chronic conditions and disabilities, contact the National Childbirth Trust, page 250.

## DIABETES

One in every 200 women has diabetes before pregnancy, this is known as diabetes mellitus. In addition, about 3 in every 100 women develop diabetes during pregnancy (called gestational diabetes). Both diabetes mellitus and gestational diabetes carry a slightly increased risk to the baby, though this risk is greatly reduced if the diabetes is well controlled.

Diabetes is a condition in which a person's pancreas gland does not produce enough insulin. Insulin is the hormone that converts the glucose (sugar) in the blood into energy for the body to use. If glucose is not converted into a usable form of energy, it builds up in the bloodstream.

During pregnancy, the level of glucose (sugar) in the mother's blood is normally raised. If, at the same time, a mother is not producing or taking enough insulin, her glucose levels become far too high and cannot be converted into the energy she needs. Although glucose can pass freely across the placenta into the baby's bloodstream, insulin cannot. If the level of glucose in the baby's bloodstream rises, the baby's pancreas gland responds by producing high levels of insulin. Since insulin also stimulates growth, the baby may become very large and will need correspondingly greater amounts of oxygen and nutrients. If the placenta cannot provide enough oxygen to meet the needs of such a large baby, he or she may die in the womb.

Babies of mothers with uncontrolled or poorly controlled diabetes mellitus are also more at risk of congenital abnormalities (see pages 201–2 and 215). This increased risk is thought to be due to high blood glucose levels during the crucial first few weeks of pregnancy while the baby's organs are developing.

Diabetic mothers may also be more vulnerable to urinary tract infections if there is a high level of glucose in their systems. This can spill over into the urine, creating a favourable environment for bacteria (see page 193). Diabetic mothers also have a higher risk of pregnancy-induced hypertension (see page 188).

Raised insulin levels in the baby's blood during pregnancy may prevent the baby's lungs from producing surfactant and may cause respiratory distress syndrome (see page 228) after delivery.

**Another pregnancy**: The increased risks to a baby if a mother has diabetes mellitus can be greatly reduced and even eradicated if the diabetes is well controlled before conception and throughout pregnancy. In addition, the baby's condition can be monitored closely and, if necessary, the baby can be delivered early by caesarean section. Standards of medical care and expertise vary a good deal and a diabetic woman who is worried about a future pregnancy, may wish to ask her GP to refer her to a specialist diabetic pre-pregnancy clinic for advice before she becomes pregnant.

In a very few cases, if a woman has diabetes mellitus with severe kidney (renal) disease and hypertension, or with severe ischaemic heart disease, the danger of pregnancy, both for her and for a baby, is very high and she may be advised not to become pregnant.

Gestational diabetes is likely to recur in future pregnancies but can be carefully watched and controlled. In women who are overweight the risk of recurrence can be reduced by losing weight before becoming pregnant again. A woman who is worried about gestational diabetes recurring may wish to ask her GP to refer her to a specialist diabetic pre-pregnancy clinic well before she becomes pregnant.

For more information about diabetes and pregnancy, contact the British Diabetic Association, see page 246.

EPILEPSY

Women with epilepsy have a very slightly increased rate of miscarriage and stillbirth and of having babies with congenital defects. Some of these risks are increased if women take anti-convulsant drugs, but giving up the drugs may cause other problems and most neurologists do not advise it.

Epileptic attacks that develop into status epilepticus (in which the fit does not stop by itself, or several fits follow in short succession without time to recover in between) may deprive a baby of oxygen in the womb and may occasionally cause miscarriage or brain damage. Very rarely, a fall during an epileptic attack can cause severe injury which can damage the baby.

All the drugs used to control epilepsy are thought to slightly increase the risk of congenital abnormalities in the baby. The most common effects of the drugs are relatively slight, and include poor growth in the womb, cleft lip and cleft palate. Very rarely anti-epileptic drugs can cause congenital heart defects and other developmental abnormalities which may be severe or fatal.

**Another pregnancy**: In planning another pregnancy it is very important to discuss the options in detail with someone with specialist knowledge, usually a neurologist. Current medical advice seems to be that, on balance, there is probably less risk to both mother and baby if the epilepsy is controlled, and if the lowest suitable dose of just one drug (rather than a combination) is taken. However, what is best for each individual will differ and must be carefully considered.

For support and advice, contact the British Epilepsy Association, see page 246.

HIGH BLOOD PRESSURE

Some women have high blood pressure (also called essential hypertension or hypertensive disease) before they become pregnant. There are thought to be many different mechanisms which combine to cause high blood pressure, most of which are not yet fully understood. High blood pressure can cause problems in pregnancy since the normal additional increased pressure caused by the extra blood in the mother's circulation due to the pregnancy may put a strain on her heart, the blood vessels leading away from the heart (arteries) and the kidneys.

In addition, whenever blood pressure rises in the body, the blood vessels automatically become narrower to cut down the excess flow of blood to the vital organs and protect them from damage. In a pregnant woman with pre-existing hypertension, the tiny blood vessels supplying the placenta may also narrow and become constricted. This can cause placental insufficiency (see page 180) and in rare cases the baby may die.

Women with pre-existing high blood pressure are more likely to develop pregnancy-induced hypertension as well (see page 188), which may also be referred to as superimposed pregnancy-induced hypertension. If this becomes severe or develops into eclampsia (see page 189), both mother and baby are at serious risk. The baby must be delivered immediately.

**Another pregnancy:** In a future pregnancy the mother's health will be carefully monitored, and the high blood pressure will be treated with bed rest and anti-hypertensive drugs. These have not been shown to have any effect on babies, but different drugs may have mild or serious temporary side-effects for the mother.

For more about high blood pressure and pregnancy, contact the British Heart Foundation, see page 246.

KIDNEY DISEASE

Women with severe pre-existing kidney conditions, such as chronic nephritis, can have increased problems during pregnancy. Their babies are also at higher risk of miscarriage, prematurity and stillbirth. The most serious problems are likely to occur if the mother develops high blood pressure during pregnancy (see Pregnancy-induced hypertension, page 188). This can damage the placenta and may cause serious, even fatal, damage to the baby.

Women with chronic kidney disease are also at increased risk of urinary tract infection (see page 194). They are more likely to go into premature labour and this can cause severe problems if the baby is very premature.

If the mother's kidneys become unable to filter off and pass toxic waste into her urine, both the baby's survival and the mother's life are at risk, and it may be necessary to deliver the baby urgently.

**Another pregnancy:** A woman with kidney disease who is

worried about a future pregnancy may wish to ask her GP to refer her to a specialist nephrologist for advice before she becomes pregnant.

For more information about kidney disease and pregnancy, contact the British Kidney Patients Association, see page 246.

## SICKLE CELL DISEASE

Sickle cell disease is an inherited blood disease that affects some people whose families originated in Africa, the Caribbean, Asia and eastern Mediterranean countries. Sickle cell disease affects the haemoglobin in the red blood cells. Haemoglobin (often written as Hb) carries oxygen all round the body, releasing it where it is needed.

Red blood cells are normally smooth and rounded, but in people with sickle cell disease they sometimes become sharp and sickle-shaped when they release oxygen. These sickle-shaped blood cells cannot flow smoothly through the very narrow blood vessels in the body. They block the circulation of the blood and cause a very painful episode called a sickle cell crisis.

There are several types of sickle cell disease, including sickle cell anaemia (often written as HbSS), SC disease (Hb SC), and sickle beta-thalassaemia (Hb S beta-thal or Hb S $\beta$-thal). All these types of sickle cell disease carry an increased risk of miscarriage and stillbirth. In women with sickle cell anaemia, which is the most serious form of sickle cell disease, the risk of losing a baby during pregnancy is roughly double the average risk in the UK.

Sickle cell disease makes people more vulnerable to infections, especially of the urinary tract (see page 194). In a pregnant woman the resulting high temperatures can cause the womb to contract and lead to premature labour. Pregnancy-induced hypertension (see page 188) is also more common. Sometimes sickling occurs in the blood vessels that lead to the placenta, cutting off some of the blood supply. If this happens, the baby may die because of lack of oxygen and nutrients. Babies of mothers with sickle cell disease are also often smaller and therefore more vulnerable after birth because of their mother's anaemia.

**Another pregnancy:** If a woman with sickle cell disease has a history of problems in pregnancy or of severe sickling, doctors may decide to try to reduce the risk to the baby in a future pregnancy by giving the mother exchange blood transfusions every few weeks throughout the pregnancy. Some of her own blood is removed and she receives blood from a donor who does not have sickle cell disease. This procedure carries certain risks for the mother, since, for example, people who have many blood transfusions may develop antibodies which make it difficult to keep finding suitable donor blood for them. However, experience in several hospitals indicates that exchange blood transfusions can reduce serious risk both to the baby and to the mother.

If a baby inherits sickle cell disease (inheriting a gene for the disease from both parents) it will not be apparent in the womb or until the baby is about 3 months old. Until that age a baby has a different kind of haemoglobin (fetal haemoglobin or Hb F) and will not be affected. If a baby is known to be at risk of inheriting sickle cell disease, a test can be carried out during pregnancy to check. This may be done by chorion villus sampling (see page 143) or, more usually, by taking a sample of the baby's blood from the umbilical cord (cordocentesis — see page 144). If the baby is found to have inherited a form of sickle cell disease the parents may be faced with the decision whether to continue the pregnancy (see also Another pregnancy, pages 138—9).

For more information about sickle cell disease and pregnancy, contact the Sickle Cell Society, see page 247.

SYSTEMIC LUPUS ERYTHEMATOSUS (LUPUS)
Systemic lupus erythematosus (lupus or SLE) is a chronic and sometimes serious multi-system inflammatory disease. It is an auto-immune disease, in which the body's immune system can turn in upon itself and attack its own connective tissues and organs. The symptoms of lupus vary a great deal. Many people have few or no symptoms; some feel ill and weak much of the time; and some develop skin rashes, aching joints, inflamed tendons and kidney problems. Lupus is most common in young women, and usually goes into remission, or at least becomes less active, after the menopause.

Women with lupus have an increased rate of miscarriage and stillbirth. At present, the reasons for this are not fully understood but research shows that some women with lupus have high levels of an antibody called anti-cardiolipin, which makes their blood more likely to clot. This can endanger a baby in the womb, since clots may form in the blood vessels leading to the placenta, cutting off the supply of oxygen and nutrients.

The causes of lupus are not yet known, though research indicates that several factors are involved, including heredity, hormones and infections. It is thought that some people inherit a tendency to develop the disease. In these people the disease may then be triggered by other factors such as physical or emotional stress, or hormonal changes in the body, for example at puberty or in the period after pregnancy. It may also follow intense exposure to the sun. Lupus cannot be cured, but most people with lupus benefit from treatment and can live a normal life.

Lupus is thought to affect one in every 1,000 people in the UK. It is more common in other countries, for example in the West Indies, parts of Asia and in North and South America. It can be detected by a simple blood test called a blood anti-nuclear antibody factor test.

**Another pregnancy:** Nowadays treatment is available during pregnancy which increases the chance that a baby will survive. A woman with lupus may wish to ask her GP to refer her to a specialist pre-pregnancy lupus clinic for counselling and advice before becoming pregnant again. If the disease is active, and particularly if it is affecting the heart, lungs or kidneys, a woman may be advised to wait until attempts have been made to control the disease before conceiving. During pregnancy, a woman with lupus may be given steroids to reduce antibody production. The pregnancy needs careful monitoring and drug levels may need frequent adjustment. A baby born to a mother with lupus has only a slightly increased risk of developing the disease.

For more information about lupus, contact Lupus UK or the adviser on lupus in the welfare department of Arthritis Care, see page 247.

## PROBLEMS TO DO WITH THE BABY'S DEVELOPMENT

Most babies who are developing abnormally are miscarried in the second or third months of pregnancy. However, some babies with life-threatening conditions or abnormalities live until late pregnancy and even beyond delivery. Although surgical and other techniques can now do a great deal, not all conditions can be corrected.

Problems in the baby's development are generally called congenital malformations, congenital abnormalities or congenital anomalies. 'Congenital' simply means something that a person is born with. It does not mean that the condition is inherited from his or her parents, though some congenital conditions are inherited. Congenital abnormalities are slightly more common if a mother is carrying two or more babies.

**Another pregnancy:** With continuing advances in medical science it is increasingly possible to diagnose congenital abnormalities and other problems while a baby is still in the womb. This may be done by alfa-fetoprotein blood tests, amniocentesis, ultrasound scan, chorion villus sampling, fetal blood sampling or other means. (For more information about these see pages 138—45.)

In a few cases it is then possible to treat the condition while the baby is still in the womb. But in most cases, treatment is still not possible, and parents whose baby is found during the pregnancy to have a serious developmental abnormality or a serious congenital illness may be faced with the decision whether to continue the pregnancy or not. Parents who are faced with this decision should be given all the information and support they need to make whatever decision is right for them. They should not be put under pressure to make their decision in a hurry.

Some parents will decide to terminate the pregnancy. Others will decide to let it take its course and to use the remaining weeks and months before the birth to prepare themselves for whatever is to come. Parents who wish to discuss the options open to them, or who would like support and advice before or after a therapeutic termination, may like to contact Support After Termination for Fetal Abnormality (SATFA) as well as any organisation that deals specifically with their baby's condition (see page 245 and pages 246—8).

We outline below the main problems to do with the baby's development that may cause death before, during or after birth.

CHROMOSOME ABNORMALITIES
Chromosomes govern what a baby inherits from his or her parents. All the cells in the human body, except the egg and sperm

cells, normally contain forty-six chromosomes, arranged in twenty-three pairs. One chromosome in each pair is inherited from the mother, and the other from the father. These chromosomes are tiny, thread-like structures in the nucleus of the cell, each made up of several thousand genes. It is through the genes that physical and certain other characteristics are passed on from parents to child. Each gene or pair of genes is responsible for certain inherited characteristics.

During the formation of egg and sperm cells, each parent's original forty-six chromosomes normally combine and divide to produce twenty-three chromosomes. At fertilisation, the twenty-three chromosomes in the sperm cell combine with the twenty-three chromosomes in the egg cell. The resulting forty-six chromosomes in the fertilised egg become the new baby's full set of chromosomes. They determine how the baby develops and form the key part of every cell in his or her body.

The process by which chromosomes combine and divide during the formation of the sperm cells and the egg cells is very complicated. If something goes wrong during this process, the fertilised egg may end up with an abnormal number of chromosomes, for example forty-five or forty-seven, or sixty-nine (a complete extra set), or with extra parts of chromosomes, or with parts of chromosomes missing or wrongly attached.

Each chromosome affects the way a baby develops from the very beginning. Most babies with abnormal chromosomes of any kind miscarry in the first few weeks. Doctors estimate that about half of all early miscarriages are due to a chromosomal abnormality which would have been incompatible with life.

Some babies with abnormal chromosomes survive to delivery, but many are born with severe abnormalities of the heart, kidneys, digestive or other organs, and may only live for a few hours or days after birth. Relatively common examples of chromosome abnormalities which usually lead to stillbirth or death within a few months of birth include: Edwards' syndrome, in which there is an extra eighteenth chromosome (also known as Trisomy 18); and Patau's syndrome, in which there is an extra thirteenth chromosome (also known as Trisomy 13). (Syndrome is the medical term for a combination of abnormal features. Trisomy means that there are three chromosomes when there should be a pair.)

There is a large number of other syndromes caused by different chromosomal abnormalities, many of which cause miscarriage, stillbirth and neonatal death. A few chromosome abnormalities, such as Down's syndrome, are not usually fatal, though babies with Down's syndrome are more likely also to have congenital defects of, for example, the heart and the gastro-intestinal system.

**The causes of chromosomal abnormalities**

In most cases, chromosomal abnormalities occur accidentally when the egg or sperm cells are forming. This is known medically as *non-disjunction*, i.e., the chromosomes simply did not separate or 'disjunct' properly during the formation of that particular egg or sperm cell. The fertilised egg that results has abnormal chromosomes. The risk of having a baby with chromosomal abnormalities due to non-disjunction increases as the mother gets get older, particularly once she is over 40.

Very occasionally, one parent (or even more rarely both parents) has an inherited tendency to produce a fairly high proportion of abnormal chromosomes, even though they themselves are unaffected. This is known medically as a *balanced chromosomal translocation*. The parent has the complete ('balanced') amount of genetic material, but it is rearranged ('translocated') among the chromosomes so that some may have too much and others may have too little. Since this parent has the complete amount of genetic material in total (though it is abnormally divided between the twenty-three pairs of chromosomes), his or her own development is unaffected. But when this parent's abnormal chromosomes divide to produce the chromosomes in the egg or sperm cells, chromosomes with too much or too little genetic material may be passed on.

Parents who are found to have a balanced chromosomal trans-location have an increased risk of chromosomal abnormalities in future pregnancies, and will be offered genetic counselling to help them make an informed choice about what to do (see pages 118–22).

**Edwards' syndrome (Trisomy 18)**

This syndrome can cause a range of abnormalities including congenital heart and kidney defects and severe mental handicap. Most babies with Edwards' syndrome miscarry or die before birth. A small number of babies with the syndrome are born alive but most of these die within the first year of life. A very small number live for several years, though many have respiratory and feeding problems in addition to those mentioned above.

**Patau's syndrome (Trisomy 13)**

Patau's syndrome can cause a range of abnormalities including severe heart, intestinal and urogenital abnormalities and severe mental handicap. Most babies with Patau's syndrome miscarry or die before birth. A small number of babies with the syndrome are born alive but most of these die within their first year. A very small number survive for several years though many have feeding and respiratory problems in addition to those mentioned above.

For information and support from other parents of babies with Edwards' syndrome, Patau's syndrome and other chromosomal abnormalities, contact the Support Organisation For Trisomy 13/18 and related disorders (SOFT UK), see page 247. For contact and support from other parents whose babies were born with other chromosome abnormalities, however rare, and even if unspecified, contact the Rare Unspecified Chromosome Disorder Support Group, see page 247.

NEURAL TUBE DEFECTS

Neural tube defects is the medical term for malformations of the spinal cord and the brain. The brain is a soft organ surrounded by membranes called meninges and enclosed within the skull. The spinal cord, also surrounded by meninges, leads out of the brain and down the spine. Both the brain and the spinal cord are bathed in cerebro-spinal fluid produced in the brain. The brain and the spinal cord (known as the central nervous system or CNS) control all the body's activities.

A developing baby's spinal cord and brain begin to form between fifteen and twenty-five days gestation and are called the neural tube. A groove forms along a flat sheet of cells which will eventually become the baby's back. The two sides of the groove then meet across the top and join to form the brain, the spinal cord and the spinal column, which protects the vulnerable spinal cord. If the two sides of the spinal column do not meet and join properly, the spinal cord may be left incompletely developed, exposed and vulnerable. The brain may also not form properly.

This causes what is called a neural tube defect, of which the main types are anencephaly and spina bifida:

## Anencephaly

This is the most severe neural tube defect. In an anencephalic baby the upper part of the brain (cerebrum) and most of the lower part (cerebellum) do not develop during the first few weeks of pregnancy. Anencephaly means 'without a brain'. The bones of the skull may also not form properly and the top of the baby's head may be misshapened.

Some babies with anencephaly miscarry. A few are stillborn, and those who are born alive die within a few hours or days of birth.

## Spina bifida

This literally means 'divided spine'. It is caused when the vertebrae in the spinal column do not close properly around the spinal cord. In severe cases, a portion of the spinal cord with nerves and the surrounding meninges grows through the gap and protrudes outside the body. (This is called a myelomeningocele.) Many babies with spina bifida also have hydrocephaly (see below) and these babies are at particular risk of death or severe handicap.

In some cases, parents and doctors may decide that the quality of life of a baby born with severe spina bifida or with spina bifida and hydrocephalus (see below) is likely to be so poor that they should not prolong it artificially by intensive medical intervention. Some babies with spina bifida miscarry during pregnancy — many during the first three months.

**Causes:** The causes of neural tube defects are not yet understood but it is now thought that both environmental and hereditary factors are involved, and that more than one gene may affect the development of the neural tube. It seems likely that some babies inherit genes that cause their neural tubes to close more slowly. It also seems that during this period, these babies are more vulnerable to something, as yet unknown, which causes neural tube defects. The most influential current theory is that certain dietary deficiencies or poor absorption by the mother or the baby of certain nutrients may contribute to the development of neural tube defects.

The risk is higher if there is a family history of neural tube defects, though between 90 and 95 per cent of babies with neural tube defects are born to parents with no family history of such defects.

**Incidence:** The rate of spina bifida and other neural tube defects varies from country to country, and also within countries. Neural tube defects are most common among white people and least common among people of African and Afro-Caribbean origin. They are more common in families of poorer social classes. The UK has a high incidence compared to other countries, even in Europe. Within the UK, neural tube defects are more common in certain areas, for example in Northern Ireland and Wales. The reason for this is unknown but heredity is thought to be a factor.

**Another pregnancy:** If parents have had one baby with a neural tube defect, there is thought to be a one in 25 chance in each future pregnancy that the baby will have either spina bifida or anencephaly. If parents have had two babies with neural tube defects, the risk for future pregnancies increases to one in 7.

Recent and continuing research suggests that improving a woman's overall diet before and during pregnancy may help to reduce the recurrence of neural tube defects. However, it is not yet known whether there are any specific nutrients which may help to prevent neural tube defects. A controlled scientific trial is in progress to try to identify the nutrients involved. This trial is particularly important since it is known that too much of certain vitamins and minerals can harm a developing baby.

Most severe neural tube defects can be detected by alpha-fetoprotein blood testing, amniocentesis and/or ultrasound scan (see pages 140–5). Sophisticated ultrasound machines may be used to assess the severity of the defect. Parents can then decide whether to terminate the pregnancy or to continue with it and use this time to prepare for an affected baby. (See also page 202 and Another Pregnancy, pages 138–9.)

For information and advice about neural tube defects and up-to-date news about current research, contact the Association for Spina Bifida and Hydrocephalus (ASBAH), see page 246.


HYDROCEPHALUS (HYDROCEPHALY)

Hydrocephalus is commonly known as water on the brain,

though the 'water' is cerebro-spinal fluid. Cerebro-spinal fluid is produced all the time from each of the four spaces (ventricles) within the brain. It normally flows from one ventricle to the next through narrow pathways, then out over the outside of the brain and down along the spinal cord. It is then absorbed into the bloodstream. If any of the drainage pathways have not developed properly or become blocked, the cerebro-spinal fluid builds up in the ventricles in the brain and causes them to swell. This puts pressure on the fragile brain tissue. The soft bones of the skull are pushed out by the pressure and the head becomes enlarged. The baby may need to be delivered by caesarean section. Some babies who develop hydrocephalus in the womb miscarry or are stillborn. Some die shortly after birth.

**Causes:** Hydrocephalus that develops in the womb can have many causes and often the cause is not known. Hydrocephalus may occur with chromosome abnormalities (see page 202) or spina bifida (see page 206). It can also be caused by an infection such as toxoplasmosis (see page 193) during the early months of pregnancy. In a very few cases, especially when hydrocephalus occurs in boys, there is a hereditary factor. Occasionally, a premature baby may develop hydrocephalus after delivery if there is severe bleeding in the brain (called intraventricular haemorrhage — see page 230). The pressure on the brain can often be relieved by inserting a small tube (known as a shunt) into the brain to drain the fluid into the abdominal cavity, though this carries some danger of infection. A shunt may also be used for a baby with congenital hydrocephalus to relieve the pressure of the cerebro-spinal fluid on the brain. In some specialist centres shunts are inserted while the baby is still in the womb.

**Another pregnancy:** The risk of hydrocephalus in future pregnancies depends on the cause of hydrocephalus in the baby who has died. In most cases there is no increased risk. Hydrocephalus can usually be detected in the womb by ultrasound scan.

For information and advice about hydrocephalus, contact the Association for Spina Bifida and Hydrocephalus (ASBAH), see page 246.

RHESUS DISEASE

Each of us has either rhesus positive or rhesus negative blood: we inherit our rhesus factor from our parents. Most people are rhesus positive. At any time during a pregnancy, small quantities of blood cells from the baby can pass accidentally into the mother's bloodstream. This is known as a feto-maternal transfusion. Sometimes there is no clear reason for it; sometimes it is due to placenta praevia (see page 183), mild placental abruption (see page 182) or some other form of bleeding in the womb, for example after amniocentesis (see page 142); and sometimes bleeding follows a miscarriage, an ectopic pregnancy or a termination. In most cases a feto-maternal transfusion causes no problems.

But if a woman with rhesus negative blood is carrying a baby with rhesus positive blood (inherited from the father — see below), she may quickly develop antibodies to her baby's rhesus positive red blood cells because her immune system perceives them as a threat. For this reason, if a mother is rhesus negative, doctors normally watch carefully for any bleeding from the baby into the mother's system. If bleeding is detected, the mother is immediately given an injection of anti-D which prevents the formation of rhesus antibodies.

However, if for some reason the blood passing from a first rhesus positive baby into a rhesus negative mother's bloodstream during pregnancy is not detected and/or anti-D is not given, the mother may develop antibodies to her baby's red blood cells. These pass into the baby's bloodstream and begin to destroy the baby's red blood cells. Red blood cells carry oxygen around the body, and in severe cases the baby becomes very short of oxygen. The heart then has to work harder to try to get enough oxygen round the body in the blood and the baby may become very anaemic (short of oxygen) and may develop heart failure (see Hydrops fetalis below) in the womb. In a very few rhesus negative women, anti-D is not effective in preventing the formation of rhesus antibodies, and the same problems may occur. Although it is rare for problems to occur in a first pregnancy with a rhesus positive baby, if they do occur they are often very serious.

Usually little or no blood passes from a baby to a mother during her first pregnancy. In this case a rhesus negative mother carrying a rhesus positive baby does not develop antibodies to this baby's blood cells. However, at delivery, when the placenta comes away from the wall of the womb, a larger amount of blood from the baby usually passes into the mother's bloodstream. If anti-D is not given at this point or does not work, the mother's blood begins to produce antibodies to rhesus positive blood which then threatens all future pregnancies with rhesus positive babies.

There are other rare blood group incompatibilities which may cause problems similar to those of rhesus disease and may sometimes result in stillbirth or neonatal death. These include Kell, Kidd and Duffy incompatibilities, and incompatibility to C and E antigens.

**Another pregnancy:** Once a mother has developed rhesus antibodies, all future pregnancies with rhesus positive babies will be affected. Anti-D cannot destroy existing antibodies, and it is ineffective once any rhesus antibodies have formed.

Whether a baby inherits rhesus negative or rhesus positive blood depends on the father's own inheritance. Each man carries two rhesus genes, one inherited from his father and one from his mother. At conception, a baby inherits one of these two. Some men carry two rhesus positive genes (and are known as homozygous): all their babies will be rhesus positive. Other men carry one rhesus positive and one rhesus negative gene (and are known as heterozygous). If the father is heterozygous, there is a one in 2 chance in each pregnancy that the baby will be rhesus positive. Parents should see a genetic counsellor to find out their situation and discuss the options for them.

In a future pregnancy the baby's blood group and the degree to which he or she is affected can be ascertained using special techniques of cordocentesis or amniocentesis (see pages 142 and 144).

If a baby is affected in a future pregnancy, all efforts will be directed at reducing the damage caused to the developing baby by rhesus antibodies. The most effective way of doing this is to give the baby transfusions of rhesus negative blood in the womb. The success of this treatment depends on how seriously the baby is affected. This can often be assessed by ultrasound scan. The aim of the treatment is to keep the baby healthy until he or she is old enough to be delivered. The delivery is often carried out a few weeks early, though premature delivery in itself increases the risk to a baby. After delivery a partial exchange transfusion may need to be given depending on the level of antibodies in the baby's blood at delivery.

For some mothers the risks to rhesus positive babies in future pregnancies may be so great that doctors recommend that future pregnancies are achieved by AID (Artificial Insemination by Donor) using sperm from a donor who is not rhesus positive. The decision to use AID can be difficult for both parents and information and support are vital.

**Hydrops fetalis**

The condition that babies with severe rhesus disease develop in the womb is known medically as hydrops fetalis. The baby becomes pale and swollen, due to severe anaemia (shortage of oxygen) and heart failure. The baby's liver and spleen also become enlarged because of the extra work created for them by the destruction of the red cells.

Babies with severe hydrops fetalis are stillborn or die soon after birth. A baby with less severe hydrops fetalis who is born alive may be treated with a small blood transfusion, followed by an exchange transfusion in which her or his own blood is replaced by donor blood containing a full complement of rhesus positive red blood cells with no rhesus negative antibodies. However this treatment is not always successful, especially if the baby is less than thirty-four weeks gestation, when the problems of prematurity are added to those of rhesus disease. At some hospitals, exchange transfusions can be given while the baby is still in the womb.

Hydrops fetalis can also have other causes, including congenital problems of the heart, kidneys and liver, and bacterial infections in the womb, for example, toxoplasmosis, cytomegalovirus, rubella (see pages 191–3), herpes (see page 232) and alpha thalassaemia major (see page 218).

CONGENITAL HEART PROBLEMS

While a baby is still in the womb, he or she gets oxygen from the mother's blood, through the placenta. A baby's circulation is therefore arranged to pump oxygenated blood from the placenta round the body and back again, and to bypass the lungs.

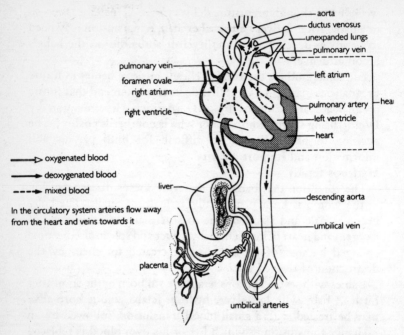

*Fig. 2* The circulation in the womb. Arrows indicate the direction of blood flow. (Adapted from J. Langman, *Medical Embryology*, 2nd Ed., Williams and Wilkins, Baltimore, 1969.)

In the womb, a temporary duct or tube (the ductus arteriosus) (see fig.2), just outside the baby's heart, connects the pulmonary artery (the artery leading to the lungs) to the aorta and diverts most of the blood in the pulmonary artery along the aorta, bypassing the lungs. There is also a small temporary valve (the foramen ovale) between the two upper chambers (atria) of the heart which allows blood to pass from the left to the right side.

As soon as a baby is born and takes the first breath, the lungs expand. There is a rush of blood from the heart to the lungs and back again. This pushes the foramen ovale closed and, within twenty-four hours, muscular activity closes the ductus arteriosus. This completely changes the baby's circulation system. The lungs are now the baby's only source of oxygen, and oxygenated blood flows all through the baby's body from the lungs.

Blood carrying oxygen now flows from the lungs through the pulmonary veins into the left atrium of the heart (see fig.3), then

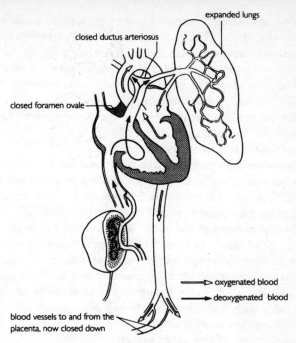

*Fig. 3* The circulation after birth.(Adapted from J. Langman, *Medical Embryology*, 2nd Ed.,Williams and Wilkins, Baltimore, 1969.)

down through a valve into the left ventricle and out into the aorta to go round the body. Deoxygenated blood (which has exchanged oxygen for carbon dioxide) comes back from the rest of the body in the two venae cavae into the right atrium of the heart. It flows down through a valve into the right ventricle and is pumped back to the lungs through the pulmonary artery to pick up oxygen again.

**What can go wrong**

If the heart has not developed properly, the baby will not be able to make the successful transition from the circulation system in the womb to that needed for survival after delivery.

The most common forms of heart malformation that can lead to neonatal death are hypoplastic left–heart syndrome, and transposition of the great arteries. These are described below. There are also many other rarer forms of heart malformation which can cause neonatal death.

In most cases, nobody knows what causes a baby's heart to

develop abnormally. Sometimes it is thought to be wholly or partly due to a chromosomal abnormality (see page 202). Sometimes there is an inherited tendency or condition carried by one or both parents (see pages 119—20). However, in most cases, no one clear cause can be found.

For support and information about congenital heart malformations, contact Heartline or the Association of Children with Heart Disorders, see pages 246—7.

**Hypoplastic left-heart syndrome**

This is the most common fatal congenital heart condition. The left ventricle of the heart does not develop properly and is very small. (Hypoplastic means underdeveloped.) As a result, very little oxygenated blood can pass from the lungs through the heart and out to the rest of the body. While the baby is in the womb this does not matter, because the baby does not depend on oxygen from its lungs. Hypoplastic left-heart syndrome therefore only begins to show when the baby is one or two days old and starts to lack oxygen. At present nothing can be done to save the life of a baby with this condition, though heart transplants may be possible in the future.

**Transposition of the great vessels**

In this condition the pulmonary artery, which carries deoxygenated blood to the lungs, and the aorta, which carries oxygenated blood round the body, are crossed over and come out of the wrong sides of the heart. This creates two completely separate circulatory systems in which the blood to and from the lungs all flows into the left-hand side of the heart. No oxygenated blood can flow to the organs in the rest of the body.

While the baby is in the womb this does not matter because the baby does not depend on oxygen from his or her lungs, and the foramen ovale and the ductus arteriosus (see above and fig. 2) allow blood to circulate around the whole circulatory system. However, once the baby is delivered and begins to breathe on its own, the foramen ovale and the ductus arteriosus close. Unless there are other ways for the blood to get through, no oxygenated blood can flow around the baby's body. In many cases, an emergency operation can now be successfully carried out to allow the baby's blood to flow around the body, but some babies with this condition still die.

**Persistent pulmonary hypertension/**
**Persistent fetal circulation**
  See page 229.

**Other congenital heart defects**
  Other dangerous congenital heart defects are:

- pulmonary valve atresia (also known as hypoplastic right-heart syndrome), in which blood flow to the baby's lungs is blocked
- tricuspid atresia, in which there is no opening to allow blood to pass through the right-hand side of the heart
- Fallot's (pronounced fallows) tetralogy, in which there is a hole in the baby's heart and also a blockage preventing blood from reaching the baby's lungs.

These and many other congenital heart defects can put a baby's life at risk. In some hospitals, some of these can now be diagnosed by detailed ultrasound scan while the baby is still in the womb. But often a severe heart defect does not become apparent until several days after the baby is born, since it takes some time for the circulatory system to finalise the changes that occur at delivery. Even in those conditions that can sometimes be successfully remedied by surgery, all operations carry some risk, especially in such tiny babies, and some babies do not survive.

  **Another pregnancy:** In most cases there is a one in 50 chance that a serious heart malformation of some kind will recur in a future pregnancy. This means that out of every 50 couples who have a baby with a serious heart condition and then go on to have another baby, one couple will have another baby with a serious heart condition. Where there is known to be an increased risk of congenital heart problems, detailed ultrasound scans will be carried out to check the baby's heart and other organs during the pregnancy.

OTHER CONGENITAL PROBLEMS
During a baby's development, problems can affect any organ. Sometimes the organ does not develop at all. Sometimes it develops only poorly, or does not work properly and so puts the baby at risk. In many individual cases, the precise cause is not understood, but known possible causes include chromosome

abnormalities (see page 202), an infection during pregnancy (see pages 190–3), environmental pollutants such as toxic metals and radiation, and medical and other drugs.

An increasing number of serious congenital malformations can now be diagnosed by ultrasound scan during pregnancy. In a few cases it is possible to undertake corrective surgery while the baby is still in the womb, though this is still very hazardous in most cases. Sometimes corrective surgery is attempted immediately after delivery. Again, the surgery itself can be very dangerous for such a small baby.

Where a serious or fatal abnormality is diagnosed during pregnancy and corrective surgery or other treatment is not possible, the parents can then decide whether to terminate the pregnancy, or whether to use the time they have to try to prepare themselves for the death of their baby soon after birth or for the care of a baby with a severe handicapping condition (see also page 202).

### Potter's syndrome

Potter's syndrome is one of several serious or fatal kidney abnormalities. In Potter's (or Potter) syndrome the baby's kidneys do not develop in the first few weeks of life in the womb. The baby's kidneys are essential for the production of amniotic fluid in the womb. If there are no kidneys, there is little or no amniotic fluid (this is known as oligohydramnios) to expand the womb around the baby and to allow the baby to grow and move. The womb remains small and in its confined space the baby's lungs cannot develop properly. Many babies with Potter's syndrome are stillborn. In those who are born alive, the immediate cause of death is failure to breathe (respiratory failure) due to underdeveloped (hypoplastic) lungs, usually one or two days after delivery. Even if this problem is treated the baby cannot survive without kidneys. (Potter's syndrome is also known as renal agenesis, which simply means that the kidneys did not develop.)

Potter's sequence is the name given to a condition which resembles Potter's syndrome in that although the baby has kidneys, there is little or no amniotic fluid (oligohydramnios). This may sometimes be because the mother's waters have broken in mid-pregnancy, or due to developmental problems in the baby's kidneys or urinary system. In Potter's sequence, as in

Potter's syndrome, the baby's lungs are compressed and cannot develop properly. The baby dies of respiratory failure within one or two days of delivery.

For contact with other parents who have experienced the syndrome, get in touch with the Potter's Syndrome Support Group, see page 247.

## TWINS AND OTHER MULTIPLE PREGNANCIES

Twin and other multiple pregnancies carry a higher risk of late miscarriage, stillbirth and neonatal death compared to single babies. This is because most complications of pregnancy are more likely with a multiple pregnancy. Mothers carrying more than one baby are more likely to go into labour prematurely, possibly because of the increased pressure of the babies on the cervix (see also Complications for premature babies, pages 226–7). In twin and other multiple pregnancies, the risk of congenital malformations (see page 211–16) is also twice as high as that for single pregnancies. Other complications more common with twins include pregnancy-induced hypertension (see page 188), anaemia and placenta praevia (see page 183).

### Twin-to-twin transfusion syndrome

Identical twins (formed from one fertilised egg) share one placenta but have two umbilical cords coming from it. In the placenta, the arteries (carrying deoxygenated blood back to the placenta) of one twin may pass very close to the veins (carrying oxygenated blood from the placenta) of the other. Occasionally they connect and blood is pumped (transfused) from one twin to the other. This deprives one twin of nutrients and haemoglobin so that she or he becomes weak, anaemic and thin. The other twin is over-supplied with blood. This twin's organs are overworked through dealing with the excess nutrients and haemoglobin, and she or he may develop heart failure and become swollen. The placenta may also be affected and may become swollen and abnormal. (This condition may also be called feto-fetal transfusion syndrome.)

Twin-to-twin transfusion syndrome can sometimes threaten the lives of both twins. More commonly, the twin who is over-supplied dies, because of the strain on her or his organs.

**Another pregnancy:** Twin-to-twin transfusion syndrome is

extremely unlikely to recur in another pregnancy. Any future twin pregnancy would be carefully watched and the babies' growth and development regularly monitored by ultrasound scan. If twin-to-twin transfusion were found the babies would be delivered as soon as it was possible for them to have a chance of survival outside the womb.

For support and contact with other parents who have lost one or both twins, contact the Twins and Multiple Births Association (TAMBA), see page 245.

## ALPHA THALASSAEMIA MAJOR

Thalassaemia is an inherited blood disorder which affects the haemoglobin in the red blood cells. Haemoglobin carries oxygen from the lungs all over the body. In each molecule of haemoglobin there is normally one pair of alpha haemoglobin chains and one pair of beta haemoglobin chains. A person who does not have all four chains may be affected with mild or severe anaemia since their blood does not contain enough haemoglobin to carry the oxygen they need around their body.

There are several forms of thalassaemia, each of different severity. Alpha thalassaemia major (sometimes written α thalassaemia major) is a very severe form in which even in the womb a baby does not make any alpha haemoglobin chains. The baby becomes very anaemic and is stillborn prematurely or dies within a few hours of birth. A baby with alpha thalassaemia major also develops hydrops fetalis (see page 211) due to severe anaemia and heart failure. Mothers whose babies have alpha thalassaemia major have an increased risk of pregnancy-induced hypertension (see page 188) and of eclampsia (see page 189).

A baby may inherit alpha thalassaemia major if both parents carry the gene that prevents the production of alpha haemoglobin. They are said to have or carry alpha thalassaemia trait (also called alpha thalassaemia minor). The trait has no symptoms. Alpha thalassaemia major occurs mainly in people whose families originated in South-East and South Asia, and occasionally in people whose families originated in the Mediterranean area.

**Another pregnancy:** If both parents carry the trait for alpha thalassaemia, each baby they have can inherit in one of three ways.

In each pregnancy:

- there is a one in 4 chance that the baby will inherit alpha thalassaemia major
- there is a one in 4 chance that the baby will inherit normal haemoglobin
- there is a 2 in 4 chance that the baby will inherit the trait for alpha thalassaemia. A baby with alpha thalassaemia trait carries the gene like his or her parents, but has no ill effects. For a diagram showing recessive inheritance see page 120.

In a future pregnancy, parents who know that they both carry the alpha thalassaemia trait may choose to have the baby's haemoglobin analysed to see what kind of haemoglobin he or she has inherited. This is done by fetal blood sampling (cordocentesis) or chorionic villus sampling (see pages 143–5). If the baby is found to have alpha thalassaemia major, which is incompatible with life, the parents may choose to terminate the pregnancy or to use the time they have to prepare themselves for the death of their baby at or soon after birth (see also page 202).

For more information about thalassaemia and pregnancy, contact the UK Thalassaemia Society, see page 248.

## PROBLEMS DURING LABOUR

Most stillborn babies have died before labour begins but a few die during labour. A death during labour may occur when the baby's oxygen supply is unexpectedly and suddenly cut off, for example by placental abruption or a prolapsed cord (see below). Or the normal physical stresses of labour may prove too much for a baby who is not strong, possibly due to congenital abnormalities (see page 201) or long-term placental insufficiency (see page 180), or because he or she is premature. Occasionally, no cause can be found for the death of a baby during labour.

For support and contact with other parents whose babies have died before or during labour, or shortly afterwards, contact the Stillbirth and Neonatal Death Society (SANDS) or one of the other bereavement support organisations listed, see pages 245–51.

## PROBLEMS TO DO WITH THE PLACENTA

### PLACENTAL ABRUPTION (ABRUPTIO PLACENTAE)

The strong contractions of the womb during labour can sometimes cause a large part of the placenta suddenly to come away from the wall of the womb. This cuts off the baby's oxygen supply and the baby may, in severe cases, die within a few minutes. Doctors normally perform an emergency caesarean section but it may be too late to save the baby.

Placental abruption in labour may be associated with pregnancy-induced hypertension (see page 188). It may also occur without any discernible cause at all. Because it happens so suddenly, there may be no way of predicting it, even with intensive monitoring. (See pages 180 and 182 for more about the placenta and for placental abruption before labour begins.)

### PLACENTAL FAILURE

A history of placental insufficiency during pregnancy (see page 180) can give rise to serious problems in labour, since the baby begins labour already weak and short of oxygen and may not be able to cope with the normal stresses of being born. This may be indicated by the slowing down of the baby's heartbeat and the baby passing meconium (waste from the baby's bowels, see also Birth asphyxia, page 222). If the baby seems to be in danger, doctors carry out a delivery as soon as possible, either by forceps or caesarean section.

## PROBLEMS TO DO WITH THE UMBILICAL CORD

The umbilical cord connects the baby to the placenta. Through the cord, the baby receives oxygen and nutrients from the mother, and passes waste products back to her. The umbilical cord is made up of two arteries and a vein, encased in a thick jelly-like substance which protects the blood vessels and stops them becoming compressed.

The baby relies on the umbilical cord for oxygen until delivery, when she or he should start to breathe air. Serious problems may occur if, for some reason, the blood vessels in the cord become blocked during delivery. All the problems described here are very rare.

PROLAPSED CORD

This occurs when the cord slips down (prolapses) into the mother's vagina during labour. This can happen if, for example, the waters have broken with a rush and the baby's head was not low down in the pelvis (engaged). There is then room for the cord to slip down through the birth canal. If a loop of the cord slips out of the birth canal, and comes into contact with the air, the jelly-like case begins to harden and the blood vessels begin to close, cutting off the baby's supply of oxygen. Unless the cord can be pushed back, and the baby delivered by caesarean section, he or she may die.

Sometimes the cord does not come right out of the birth canal but slips down beside the baby's head. This can happen even if the waters have not broken. As the baby passes through the birth canal, the cord is squeezed between the baby's head and the mother's pelvic bone, especially during contractions. This is difficult to detect unless the cord can be felt, though changes in the heartbeat will probably alert staff to the problem. The baby becomes increasingly short of oxygen and may die unless an emergency caesarean is carried out in time. A prolapsed cord is more common if the baby is in the breech position.

TRUE KNOT

This condition is called a true knot to distinguish it from false knots which are bulges in the cord. A true knot occurs when the umbilical cord knots while the baby moves about in the womb. During delivery, the cord may stretch and pull the knot tight and it has long been thought that this cuts off the baby's oxygen supply and causes death. However, the umbilical cord is strong and is well protected by the jelly-like substance that surrounds it and by the pressure of the blood inside it. It seems more likely therefore that in most cases a true knot only pulls tight after the baby has died and the blood pressure in the cord has fallen and the cord lost its tension. In most cases, the death itself cannot be explained in the light of current medical knowledge.

CORD AROUND THE NECK

The discovery of the cord around the neck of a baby who has died is fairly common. However, as with a true knot (see above), it is now thought that this is very rarely the cause of a baby's death, and in most cases the baby has died from another, often unknown, cause.

As a baby moves and turns in the womb, the umbilical cord often becomes wrapped around the baby's neck or body. In a healthy baby this is unlikely to cause damage. The cord is usually too strong to become stretched so thin that it cuts off the supply of oxygen to the baby. Even if the cord is around the baby's neck this should not cause damage since in the womb a baby does not breathe through his or her windpipe. It seems likely that in most cases where a baby is born dead and the umbilical cord is found to be tightly round the body or neck, the tightening occurred after the baby died when the cord had lost its tension and elasticity. In most cases the death itself cannot be explained in the light of current medical knowledge.

## BIRTH ASPHYXIA

### FETAL DISTRESS

The medical term 'fetal distress' means that too little oxygen is passing through the placenta into the baby's bloodstream during labour. This may happen if:

- the labour is very long
- the contractions of the womb (which temporarily obstruct the oxygen supply to the placenta) are very frequent
- the baby's oxygen supply is cut off as a result of problems with the cord (see page 220) or because of placental abruption (see page 220)
- if the baby is fragile because of previous growth or other problems.

Fetal distress means a lack of oxygen in the bloodstream. The most likely effect on the baby is that he or she becomes drowsy and later unconscious. It does not mean that the baby is distressed or in pain.

If a baby becomes 'distressed' during delivery or at any other time, the baby's body responds by concentrating blood flow to the brain and heart, which are the most important organs for survival. Blood flow to other areas decreases and muscles in these areas relax. This allows the meconium (waste from the baby's bowel) in the baby's bowel to pass into the amniotic fluid. The sight of blackish-green meconium in the mother's waters alerts midwives and doctors to the fact that something may be wrong. But passing meconium is not always a sign of distress and is often the response of a mature baby to the normal stress of labour. (See below for more about risks caused by meconium.) Other signs of fetal distress in labour are a persistent slow or fast heart rate.

Severe fetal distress, that is, severe lack of oxygen, may result in the death of a baby during or immediately after delivery. Monitoring cannot always detect fetal distress in time to prevent death or severe handicap.

MECONIUM ASPIRATION

If there is meconium (waste from the baby's bowels — see above) in the amniotic fluid, the baby may breathe it (aspirate it) into her or his lungs. This is most likely to occur when a baby is short of oxygen during labour (see Fetal distress, page 222) or at delivery (known as birth asphyxia). Meconium in the baby's lungs blocks the thin cell walls and prevents oxygen passing through them into the bloodstream. Meconium also irritates the lining of the lungs and can cause an inflammation known as chemical pneumonitis.

Meconium aspiration is most likely at the time of delivery as the baby takes his or her first full breath of air. The meconium may then be breathed right into the lungs. But if a baby has passed meconium earlier, aspiration can also occur earlier in labour or, rarely, before labour begins. Babies in the womb practice breathing movements. If a baby becomes short of oxygen in the womb, she or he may make reflex breathing or gasping movements which increase the risk of taking in meconium.

In some cases, a baby with meconium aspiration goes on to develop pneumothorax, a dangerous condition in which a hole develops in the lung, and air escapes through it into the chest. This air then exerts pressure on the lungs and prevents them expanding. The group of problems that can arise after a baby has breathed in meconium during labour are known by the collective name meconium aspiration syndrome.

Babies most at risk of meconium aspiration syndrome are those who are born after forty-two weeks gestation (post term), who are small for dates or who have been very short of oxygen during or before labour. Babies who develop an infection in the womb such as listeriosis (see page 191), may also pass meconium before delivery and may take it in before or during delivery.

BABIES WHO DO NOT BREATHE

Sometimes a baby is too ill to breathe after delivery. This most commonly follows fetal distress in labour (see page 222). But in some cases there seems to be no reason why the baby does not breathe. These cases are impossible to predict, even with intensive monitoring during labour, though afterwards doctors may deduce that the baby has been short of oxygen at some point. Prolonged lack of oxygen to the brain depresses the baby's reflexes so that normally automatic actions like breathing may not happen.

Doctors usually try to resuscitate a baby who is not breathing, but if the baby has been deprived of oxygen for a long time he or she may die or become severely brain damaged. If resuscitation is successful, the baby may be put on a ventilator which will breathe artificially for twenty-four or forty-eight hours to see if she or he recovers and begins to breathe naturally. If not, parents and doctors have to face the difficult decision of when to stop ventilation and allow the baby to die.

# PROBLEMS AFTER BIRTH

Problems after birth may arise as a result of congenital abnormalities, problems in the supply of oxygen and nutrients to the baby during pregnancy, infections caught in the womb or during or after delivery, events during labour and delivery, or prematurity.

## PREMATURE BABIES

In the UK about 7 out of every 100 pregnancies ends in a premature birth (birth before thirty-seven weeks gestation). This rate has remained unchanged despite intensive study and concern. The survival rate of premature babies has improved tremendously in recent years, but there are still many babies who die because they are born before their systems can cope with life outside the womb. Sometimes these babies also have congenital malformations that make it impossible for them to survive.

At present, almost all babies born before twenty-six weeks, and many born before thirty weeks, die from complications of prematurity. Babies born after thirty weeks gestation are also at risk if the problems of prematurity are compounded by those of congenital abnormality, or if they become distressed (see page 222) during labour or develop an infection.

## CAUSES OF PREMATURE LABOUR
### Spontaneous premature labour
In most cases premature labour starts by itself (known medically as 'spontaneous'). If the pregnancy is less than about thirty-two weeks and the mother's health is not at risk, doctors may try to stop the labour (although hospital policies vary on this). However, current methods of delaying labour are not very effective and in most cases it is not possible to delay it for very long.

At present, the main methods of trying to stop labour are by giving a drip or tablets containing hormones (betamimetic drugs) to relax the womb. It is not thought that these affect the baby. They may temporarily make the mother's heart beat a little faster and give her a slight tremor. Doctors may also inject the mother with corticosteroids. These pass through the placenta to the baby and have been shown to speed up the development of the baby's lungs and so help prevent breathing difficulties in premature babies (see Respiratory distress syndrome, page 228).

It is not always clear why a labour has started prematurely. The main known causes of premature labour are:

- the waters breaking early (spontaneous premature rupture of the membranes) possibly due to infection (see page 190) or other causes
- multiple pregnancies, that is, where the mother is carrying two or more babies. Nearly half of all multiple pregnancies end with spontaneous premature labour and delivery, most commonly at thirty-two to thirty-four weeks gestation.
- placental abruption (see page 182)

- a weak cervix (see page 185)
- a fibroid in the womb (see page 186)
- an abnormally shaped womb (see page 187)
- a baby with severe congenital abnormalities (see page 201)
- the mother having a high temperature (see page 190)
- a urinary tract or other infection in the mother (see page 193).

A woman may also be more likely to go into spontaneous premature labour if her previous pregnancy ended prematurely, but this depends on the reason for the previous premature labour.

### Elective premature delivery

In some cases doctors decide to end a pregnancy and deliver a baby prematurely to try to save his or her life and often that of the mother as well. The main indications for this (known as an elective delivery) are:

- severe pregnancy-induced hypertension (see page 188)
- spontaneous premature rupture of the membranes which is not followed by labour within a relatively short period, especially if there are signs of an infection in the mother or the baby. (Each hospital has its own policy on when labour should be induced, but most feel that after twenty-four hours the risk of infection in the baby increases.)
- fetal distress (see page 222)
- poor fetal growth (see page 180)
- kidney disease in the mother (see page 198)
- placental abruption (see page 182)
- placenta praevia (see page 183)
- rhesus incompatibility (see page 209).

COMPLICATIONS FOR PREMATURE BABIES

The more premature a baby is at delivery, the less her or his systems are able to take on the various functions necessary for life outside the womb. Prematurity is the single most common cause of death of babies in the first week of life. Premature babies are at particular risk of complications such as:

- respiratory distress syndrome due to immature lungs (see page 228)

- bleeding of the fragile blood vessels in the brain (intraventricular haemorrhage – see page 230)
- infections. Their immune systems are immature and they may be overwhelmed by an infection very quickly (see page 230).

Premature babies are at increased risk if they are also small for their gestational age (small for dates).

No one knows why some premature babies die and others survive. Some babies seem well at birth but then become very ill. Because their systems are so small and fragile, premature babies can go through several rapid ups and downs, recovering and becoming ill again extremely fast.

In some ways choices and decisions about the care of premature babies have been made more difficult by rapid technological innovations in neonatal care. Doctors and parents may feel that it is worth trying to treat and save many babies for whom twenty years ago there would have been no hope. Although many more babies can now be saved, some still die even after intensive treatment. Improved technology has also meant that some severely handicapped babies can be kept alive when their quality of life is likely always to be poor. Parents and doctors may decide that they should not carry out intensive and often invasive treatment to keep such a baby alive. This can be an extremely difficult and distressing decision.

Many hospital neonatal units have their own support groups for parents whose babies have died. Parents of babies who have died while in a neonatal unit or shortly afterwards may like to contact SANDS (the Stillbirth and Neonatal Death Society), the bereavement group of NIPPERS (National Information for Parents of Prematures, Resources and Support) and/or BLISSLINK, see pages 245 and 250–1.

## PROBLEMS TO DO WITH THE BABY'S LUNGS

The lungs consist of thousands of tiny hollow sacs called alveoli. It is through these sacs the oxygen which has been breathed into the body passes into the bloodstream, and carbon dioxide passes back to be breathed out. Breathing (respiratory) problems are the most common cause of serious illness and death in premature babies.

## RESPIRATORY DISTRESS SYNDROME

Respiratory distress syndrome (RDS) is the term used to describe breathing problems in newborn and, especially, premature babies.

In premature babies, RDS is usually caused by a lack of surfactant in the lungs. Surfactant is a greasy liquid which prevents the alveoli (hollow sacs) in the lungs collapsing and sticking together every time the baby breathes out. A baby's lungs only produce surfactant towards the end of pregnancy. So, in babies born before about thirty-four weeks there may be too little surfactant. The alveoli and the lungs collapse and become stiff and stick together at each out-breath and it is difficult or impossible for the baby to expand his or her lungs and breathe in more oxygen. A common and dangerous complication of RDS is bleeding in the brain (intraventricular haemorrhage — see page 230).

The more premature a baby is the more she or he is at risk of RDS caused by a lack of surfactant in the lungs. RDS is also more likely if a baby has been short of oxygen during labour, since lack of oxygen slows down the production of surfactant.

Babies with severe respiratory distress syndrome may be put on a ventilator which 'breathes' for them and may give their lungs and other systems time to mature. Despite this, in some very premature babies the lungs may still be too small to allow enough oxygen to pass into the blood. Other complications may also cause respiratory distress syndrome and may be fatal. The most common are pneumonia, an infection in the lung (see below) and pneumothorax, found mainly in babies on ventilators, when a hole develops in the lung through which air escapes into the chest.

Respiratory distress syndrome caused by a lack of surfactant may also be referred to, especially in post-mortem reports, as hyaline membrane disease.

## PNEUMONIA

Pneumonia is an infection of the tiny hollow sacs in the lungs (alveoli — see above). If a baby has pneumonia, the infection causes these sacs to become filled with fluid so that oxygen cannot pass through them into the baby's bloodstream.

In newborn babies, pneumonia is usually caused by an infection caught in the womb or during delivery (see pages 190 and 230).

Premature babies who are on a ventilator for some time are also at increased risk of infection leading to pneumonia.

Pneumonia — known as chemical pneumonitis — can also occur if a baby inhales meconium (waste from the baby's bowels) during delivery (see page 223).

## PERSISTENT PULMONARY HYPERTENSION/PERSISTENT FETAL CIRCULATION

This means, literally, persistent high blood pressure in the lungs. While a baby is in the womb, the pressure on the blood vessels in the lungs is high and the vessels are narrow. Once the baby is delivered and takes his or her first breath, filling the lungs with air, pressure in the blood vessels should fall and the vessels should expand, so that blood from the heart can flow into them. The changes in pressure and the new pattern of blood circulation should cause the two ducts, the ductus arteriosus and the foramen ovale, to close (see also fig. 3 and pages 211–3).

If, for some reason, the pressure in the blood vessels of the lungs does not fall, too little blood flows to them. The foramen ovale is not pushed shut but continues to allow blood to flow from the right to the left side of the baby's heart as it did in the womb. As a result, much of the blood bypasses the pulmonary artery and does not travel to the lungs to pick up oxygen for the rest of the body. Unless the condition can be corrected by drugs or surgery, the baby becomes increasingly ill and short of oxygen, and is likely to develop heart failure.

The reasons for pulmonary hypertension are not fully understood but it often occurs in babies who have had severe meconium aspiration (see page 223). Persistent pulmonary hypertension also occurs in babies with other serious problems, such as severe respiratory distress syndrome (see page 228), a severe infection or a severe shortage of oxygen at delivery (birth asphyxia).

## BRONCHOPULMONARY DYSPLASIA

This is a serious complication in babies who have been on artificial ventilation for long periods or who have needed prolonged treatment with oxygen. The lungs and the bronchial tubes inside the lungs develop abnormally (known medically as dysplasia). The alveoli in the lungs (see page 227) become enlarged and damaged, and the lungs become scarred and less efficient at allowing oxygen to pass through into the baby's bloodstream. The heart then has to work harder to pump oxygen round the body and may fail.

Doctors now think that bronchopulmonary dysplasia may be caused by the pressure effects of artificial ventilation on the lung (some pressure is needed to prevent the lungs collapsing) and try to use the lowest pressure possible. But bronchopulmonary dysplasia is still a serious and sometimes fatal complication in some ventilated babies, especially if they are very premature.

## INTRAVENTRICULAR HAEMORRHAGE

Inside the brain there are spaces (ventricles) filled with cerebro-spinal fluid (see pages 207—8 for more about the brain). In some babies the changes of pressure during delivery can cause the blood vessels in the brain to bleed into the central ventricles and sometimes into the brain tissue itself, which can cause severe damage. Intraventricular haemorrhage (bleeding within the ventricles) is most common in babies born before thirty-three weeks gestation. The more premature the baby, the more fragile are all her or his organs and the more damage can be done.

The causes of intraventricular haemorrhage (IVH) are not yet fully understood. Some degree of IVH occurs in about 50 per cent of premature babies; this is probably due to increases in blood flow to the brain when the blood pressure goes up in the rest of the body. A baby is more susceptible to IVH if she or he gets too little oxygen during delivery. About one in 10 cases of intraventricular haemorrhage causes brain damage or death. IVH is also a common complication of respiratory distress syndrome (see page 228) and in babies with RDS, it is the most common cause of death.

If bleeding in the brain blocks the passage of cerebro-spinal fluid, the resulting pressure may cause the skull to expand leading to hydrocephalus (see page 207).

## INFECTIONS

A newborn baby may acquire an infection in the womb, in the birth canal during delivery, or after delivery. During pregnancy, and particularly towards the end, antibodies from the mother cross the placenta into the baby's bloodstream. These protect the baby against most of the bacteria and viruses the mother has already encountered and developed immunity against. However, some of the mother's antibodies are too large to cross the placenta, and all babies are therefore vulnerable to infection by certain organisms.

A newborn baby with an infection is at serious risk since his or her immune system is immature and finds it difficult to fight off any infection. Babies still in the womb and premature babies are particularly at risk since they have received fewer of their mother's antibodies and their immune systems are still more poorly developed.

Most of the infections described below are fairly rare and not much is known about them. New information is emerging all the time and there may be medical differences of opinion in some cases about how they are caught, and about treatment, diagnosis, prevention and so on.

ORGANISMS THAT CAN INFECT BABIES AT THE TIME OF DELIVERY

Many organisms live normally in the mother's vagina or back passage (rectum) and may cause no symptoms. Often the mother has not developed antibodies to these organisms to pass on to her baby as they are not physically inside her blood circulation and other systems. Some of these organisms can infect the baby just before or during delivery.

The risk of infection during delivery increases if a long period passes between the rupturing of the mother's membranes and the beginning of labour, since once the membranes have broken there is no barrier to stop the infection travelling into the womb. If this does happen, the mother may develop an infection of the membranes lining the womb (amnionitis), and sometimes an infection of the placenta (placentitis). The baby may develop blood poisoning (septicaemia) or an infection in the lungs (pneumonia), both of which can be fatal (see also below).

**Group B streptococcus**

This is the most common and important cause of fatal infection in newborn babies. It can cause septicaemia, pneumonia and, rarely, meningitis. Between 10 and 30 per cent of all women carry Group B streptococcus in their back passage (rectum) or vagina all the time, usually without any symptoms. The bacteria may reach the baby during or just before, delivery. Not all of those babies who come into contact with Group B streptococcus become infected.

Babies who are premature or small for their gestational age (sometimes called small for dates), and other babies with lowered immunity, are most vulnerable to infection. An infected baby may be born completely healthy but may become severely ill very rapidly after some hours or days.

**Another pregnancy:** Group B streptococcus can recur and cause problems in future pregnancies though this is very rare. If there is a known risk of this in a future pregnancy, great care is taken to test for the bacteria and to treat it with penicillin if necessary.

### Herpes

This virus is most dangerous if the mother has only just contracted herpes (known as a primary infection) and if the baby is delivered when the mother still has open sores (lesions) which shed the virus. Genital herpes is usually sexually transmitted. Cold sores from the mouth and whitlows on the fingers can also affect the genital area and infect the baby.

A baby infected by herpes during labour may develop a fatal infection, particularly of the brain and the meninges, the membranes surrounding the brain. The baby may also develop hydrops fetalis (see page 211). Genital herpes can also cause premature labour (see page 225).

**Another pregnancy:** The chance of a baby becoming infected with herpes is much lower in women who have recurrent genital herpes from a previous infection. In a future pregnancy, if the disease is active when the baby is due, that is, if open sores can be seen or there is other evidence of current infection, the baby will normally be delivered by caesarean section to prevent infection. There is otherwise no reason to deliver the baby by caesarean section.

For more information and support, contact the Herpes Association, see page 247.

**Listeriosis**

See page 191.

**Chicken pox (varicella zoster)**

This can cause severe and often fatal illness in a baby if the mother develops the chicken pox rash less than five days before delivery. There is then no time for her to develop antibodies and pass them on to her baby. The baby becomes infected with chicken pox through the placenta; this may lead to meningitis (see below), or encephalitis (an infection of the brain).

SECONDARY INFECTIONS

An infection may be caused in the womb or after delivery by any of the organisms listed above, and also by others, such as other streptococcal bacteria, staphylococcal bacteria, coliform bacteria and by certain viruses. An infection most often begins as pneumonia, though meningitis, septicaemia (see below) and other infections are common. Any infection can spread very quickly through the baby's body because it is small and the baby's immune systems are immature. Premature babies on ventilators, with drips and other equipment attached to their bodies, are at increased risk of infection because of the invasive procedures which they undergo.

A baby with an infection may become lethargic, reluctant to feed, may lose weight or just collapse. (Babies with even severe infections do not always develop a high temperature.) In very small and premature babies, or those who are ill already, it may be very difficult to discover the cause of these symptoms. Sometimes an infection can only be diagnosed at the post-mortem examination after the baby has died.

**Meningitis**

Meningitis is an infection of the meninges, the membranes which surround the brain. It can lead to an infection of the brain itself and to septicaemia (see below). Meningitis is extremely dangerous to a small baby and is often fatal.

**Pneumonia**

See page 228.

**Septicaemia (blood poisoning)**

Septicaemia can arise when bacteria infect a particular area and then divide rapidly and spread in the blood throughout the baby's circulatory system. The bacteria produce poisons (toxins) and cause an overwhelming infection in the whole body so that the blood vessels collapse, blood pressure falls and the heart has to work extremely hard to move the blood round the body and may fail. This is known medically as septicaemic shock.

## NECROTISING ENTEROCOLITIS

Enterocolitis is the medical term for an inflammation affecting the large and small intestine. Necrotising enterocolitis (NEC) is an inflammation of the walls of the large and small intestines which can lead to small sections of tissue dying (necrotising). It occurs mainly in newborn babies who are already vulnerable, possibly because they are very premature, weighed less than 2,000g at birth, suffered birth asphyxia (see page 222) or have respiratory distress syndrome (see page 228), septicaemia (see above), too little sugar in the blood (hypoglycaemia) or congenital heart disease (see page 211).

Necrotising enterocolitis can develop when, for any reason, the blood supply to the intestines is reduced. This causes the wall of the intestine to swell and become ulcerated. It is then vulnerable to infection, inflammation and destruction. The baby's stomach becomes swollen and the intestine may become perforated. A serious infection may lead to shock and can be fatal.

If the intestine is perforated or there is severe bleeding and medical treatment is not helping, doctors may decide to operate urgently to try to mend the damage, though this is not always successful.

# APPENDIX 2
# Principles of Good Practice

(These 'Principles of Good Practice' are taken from *Miscarriage, Stillbirth and Neonatal Death: Guidelines for Professionals*, published in 1991 by the Stillbirth and Neonatal Death Society, London. The *Guidelines* provide detailed guidance on the management of miscarriage, stillbirth and neonatal death for all professionals who come into contact with bereaved parents.)

## 1. The care given to parents should be responsive to their individual feelings and needs.

All those who are bereaved by the loss of a baby have experiences and feelings in common. But however much is shared, bereavement and grief are also intensely individual, so while it is helpful if professionals recognise and understand common patterns in parents' experiences, the care and support which they give should be determined by parents' particular needs.

It is necessary:

- to avoid assumptions
- to listen and respond to each parent as an individual
- to take account of particular circumstances, particular feelings and beliefs, and particular experiences
- to tailor what is said and what is done to the parents/family concerned
- not to be judgmental.

Many parents will be very confused about their feelings and uncertain about what they need. They need an environment where they can discover for themselves what they feel, and where their feelings are accepted. They need to be helped to work out for themselves what their loss means to them. This process may take a long time and cannot be hurried, so the care parents are given should not pressurise them. Professionals must be prepared to work flexibly, and to the parents' time-scale.

Professionals must also be prepared to accept that there may be much that parents cannot or do not want to express about the way they feel, and much that an outsider may not be able to understand. This means that it is often necessary to work with uncertainty and to risk making mistakes. What professionals offer will not always be welcomed by or be right for the parents concerned, and although it is difficult, professionals need to be able to tolerate this.

They should be aware that some parents may have special needs. The loss of a baby may, for example, be particularly traumatic for those who have fertility problems, those who have had recurrent losses, those who can have no more children or for parents of twins where one twin has died.

## 2. Parents need information.

At every stage, parents need and should be given information which is accurate and which is communicated clearly, sensitively and promptly.

In order that they can begin to understand and own their experience, parents need information:

- about what has happened, what is happening or what may happen to them
- about practical matters, procedures and arrangements
- about the choices which are open to them. They also need clear, factual, unbiased information so that they can make those choices.

It is likely that both parents will need information and it is usually best if it is given to both together. Information may be supplied in response to questions. No question should be left unanswered. If the answer is difficult for some reason, or even unknown, it is better to admit the difficulty than to ignore the question. But parents may also find it hard to put questions into words, or may not know what to ask, so it is helpful to offer information or discussion when the time seems right to do so. Offers should be repeated. No subject should be avoided. Parents need and appreciate honesty, even if the truth is painful.

It is often hard for parents to take in information the first time it is given to them; for this reason, or for other reasons, they may wish to go over it again, and even a number of times. Information should also be available in written form — not as a substitute for discussion but to back it up.

If parents speak little or no English, it is important that they are not denied information for that reason. Interpreters and written information in their own language will be needed.

All professionals in contact with the parents should give consistent information. Parents should not be confused or overwhelmed by being given information by too many different professionals. Co-ordination is important.

Information may also be needed by other family members. But parents' permission should always be asked for before talking with others.

### 3. Communication with parents should be clear, sensitive and honest.

It is essential that professionals are able to communicate with parents in ways which the parents find acceptable and supportive.

It is helpful if professionals are able:

- to set aside their professional authority when necessary and show a human face
- to talk with parents on equal terms — for example, sitting not standing, and not hiding their own grief about what has happened. Important discussions should not be held while a woman is lying down, unless this really cannot be avoided.
- to use language which is clear, caring and easy to understand. It is important to consider the meaning of words for parents and to avoid unnecessary medical jargon. This means, for example, speaking of a 'miscarriage', never of an 'abortion', and referring to the baby as a 'baby', not a 'foetus', no matter how small it is. Instead of talking about the 'disposal' of a pre-viable baby, staff might talk about 'what will be done with the baby's body'.
- to be open and honest. Parents would rather know the truth

than feel that information is being withheld from them or misrepresented. It is particularly important not to hold discussions in parents' presence which are not shared with them.

- to make time (and show that there is time) for lengthy and unhurried conversations when needed. Even if a conversation has to be postponed, parents will be helped if a firm promise is made to talk later.
- to recognise when a parent does or does not wish to talk.

When the parents do not speak English and the professional concerned is unable to speak fluently in the parents' own language, it is essential that an interpreter is used.

### 4. Parents should be treated with respect and dignity.

Parents need respect for themselves, for what they have experienced and are experiencing, and for their feelings. Their dignity is extremely important at a time when they are vulnerable. This applies equally to both parents: the father as well as the mother.

Demonstrating respect involves:

- recognising the significance of what has happened and therefore not minimising it (for example, not saying 'You can always have another baby')
- caring for parents in a way which does not deprive them of dignity. (It is particularly important to recognise that many women find gynaecological procedures both undignified and distressing. Everything possible should be done to minimise this additional distress. For example, women should not be left in the lithotomy position any longer than necessary.)
- treating and speaking about what has been lost, whether a baby, a foetus or products of conception, in a respectful way
- recognising the personal and private nature of grief by caring in a non-intrusive way and giving parents the privacy they need. For many parents, a hospital is an inappropriately impersonal and public place in which to grieve.
- enabling parents to participate in the management of their loss.

At a time when much is beyond their control, parents need to feel that they have some power over what is happening to them. They should be helped to feel in touch with and in charge of their own experience.

## 5. Parents' loss should be recognised and acknowledged, their experience and feelings validated.

Parents need others to recognise and acknowledge their loss as part of the difficult process of accepting what has happened. This need, like grief itself, continues over a long period of time.

The expression of sympathy is one important and very simple form of acknowledgement. Neither this nor other ways of acknowledging loss should be omitted because they are painful (although they undoubtedly are). It is more difficult for parents to accept what has happened if people around them appear to deny it.

Parents may also need confirmation of the reality of their experience and reassurance about their responses to it. The loss of a baby at any stage is bewildering and shocking. Parents may struggle to grasp the significance of their experience, to make sense of it in their own terms, and to accept that their feelings are legitimate. Talking about what has happened, going through both the events and the feelings, can be very important. Professionals should make themselves available to help parents do this.

Parents may also need support to do things which will make their experience real to them and create memories for the future.

## 6. Parents need to be given time.

The loss of a baby, whether as a miscarriage, stillbirth or neonatal death, often happens with an intensity and speed which makes it difficult for the experience to be grasped and understood. In the days, weeks and months afterwards, parents need to overcome shock, understand the experience they have had and begin to grieve.

Parents need:

- time with each other and/or with their family
- time, if wanted, with their baby
- time to consider and make decisions about practical arrangements

- time in which to re-live, think and talk about what has happened.

Only a very few procedures after a baby's death have to be carried out within a certain time limit (the post-mortem examination, for example, and registration). These should be explained. Parents can then be reassured that there is no other time pressure.

Professionals should try to work to the time-scale dictated by parents' feelings and needs. Some parents, for example, who do not wish to see and hold their baby at first, may want to do so later. They may find that they wish to leave hospital earlier than they had thought, or later.

Sometimes, however, it can be helpful to set time limits for certain decisions. When there is no time limit at all, some decisions (about the baby's burial or cremation, for example) can become much harder to make.

## 7. All those involved in the care of bereaved parents should be well informed.

Professionals who are in close contact with bereaved parents and are responsible for their care need to be well informed. They may need to acquire knowledge which is outside their own specific area of expertise.

Professionals need to know:

- their own hospital/community policy regarding the management of miscarriage, stillbirth and neonatal death
- about statutory procedures and practical arrangements
- about what services and support are available to parents locally
- about grief and grieving, particularly in relation to miscarriage, stillbirth and neonatal death.

They need this knowledge in order to give accurate and comprehensive information to parents, since only then can parents make informed choices. To be well informed is also important from the professional's own point of view. Few of those working with bereaved parents have extensive experience of bereavement, and for this and other reasons, many do not feel confident. Knowledge can help to give confidence.

Managers should be aware that a range of other staff will come into contact with parents, such as nursing auxiliaries, ward clerks, domestic staff, porters and receptionists. It is important that they too are informed about policy and good practice.

## 8. All those who care for and support bereaved parents should have access to support for themselves.

Professionals whose job it is to care for and support bereaved parents are likely to need support themselves. They too may be very shocked by a baby's death and may need to grieve; they may feel responsible; they may feel unable to cope with either the practical tasks involved or the emotional caring demanded of them. They may find it difficult to manage their personal reactions at the same time as performing a professional role — particularly because the event may bring up emotions to do with their own experiences of loss and bereavement.

The stress involved in the care of bereaved parents is lessened if the professionals concerned:

- receive recognition that their work is demanding and difficult and that they therefore need support, not because of professional inadequacy or personal weakness but as a necessity
- have received appropriate training
- are working within the framework of a clear operational policy
- feel confident that what they are doing or being asked to do is appropriate
- are able to work in co-operation with other professionals
- are given opportunities to explore, understand and express their own feelings — both about bereavement and grief in general and also in relation to specific cases in which they are involved.

Not all professionals will need the same kind or same degree of support. Different options should be available.

# Further Reading

Murray Enkin, Marc J. Keirse and Iain Chalmers, *A Guide to Effective Care in Pregnancy and Childbirth*, Oxford University Press, Oxford, 1989.

Valerie Hey, Catherine Itzin, Lesley Saunders and Mary Anne Speakman (eds), *Hidden Loss: Miscarriage and Ectopic Pregnancy*, The Women's Press, London, 1989.

Susan Hill, *Family*, Penguin, Harmondsworth, 1990.

Christine Moulder, *Miscarriage: Women's Experiences and Needs*, Pandora, London, 1990.

Kathy Nairne and Gerrilyn Smith, *Dealing with Depression*, The Women's Press, London, 1983.

Ann Oakley, Ann McPherson and Helen Roberts, *Miscarriage*, Penguin, Harmondsworth, 1990.

Angela Phillips and Jill Rakusen, *The New Our Bodies, Ourselves*, Penguin, Harmondsworth, 1989 (revised edition).

Mary Pipes, *Understanding Abortion*, The Women's Press, London, 1986.

Stillbirth and Neonatal Death Society, *Miscarriage, Stillbirth and Neonatal Death: Guidelines for Professionals*, London, 1991.

Rosemary Wells, *Helping Children Cope with Grief*, Sheldon Press, London, 1988.

J. Wiliam Worden, *Grief Counselling and Grief Therapy*, Tavistock/Routledge, 1991 (second edition).

# Useful Addresses

The organisations listed here vary a good deal: some are very large, some are tiny; some are run by professionals, others by parents; some have local contacts or support groups. They all welcome contact and enquiries from parents and others. It is usually a good idea to include a stamped addressed envelope.

## SUPPORT FOR PARENTS WHO HAVE LOST A BABY

**BLISSLINK**
17 – 21 Emerald Street, London WC1N 3QL (071 831 9393/8996). For parents of babies in intensive care and special care including bereaved parents.

**Foundation for the Study of Infant Deaths (FSID)**
35 Belgrave Square, London SW1X 8QB (071 235 0965). For parents whose babies have died as a result of Sudden Infant Death Syndrome (cot death or SIDS).

**Miscarriage Association (MA)**
c/o Clayton Hospital, Northgate, Wakefield, W. Yorks WF1 3JS (most weekday mornings: 0924 200799). For parents who have experienced miscarriage.

**Scottish Cot Deaths Trust**
c/o Royal Hospital for Sick Children, Yorkhill, Glasgow G3 8SJ (041 357 3946).

**NIPPERS Bereavement Group**
Janet Palmer, PO Box 1553, Wedmore, Somerset BS28 4AH (0934 733123). For bereaved parents of premature babies and babies in intensive and special care.

**Stillbirth and Neonatal Death Society (SANDS)** 0171 436 5881
28 Portland Place, London W1N 4DE (071 436 5881). For parents whose babies are born dead or who die shortly after birth. 0171 436 7940 *

**Support After Termination For Abnormality (SATFA)**
29 – 30 Soho Square, London W1V 6JB (071 439 6124). For parents who have had or may have a pregnancy terminated because of their baby's abnormality.

**Twin & Multiple Births Association (TAMBA)** (Bereavememt Support Group)
Contact through SANDS (see above). For parents who have lost one or both twins, or babies from a multiple birth.

## ORGANISATIONS LINKED TO SPECIFIC MEDICAL CONDITIONS

**Association of Children with Heart Disorders**

17 Cole Lane, Mossley, Ashton-under-Lyme, Lancashire OL5 9DS (0457 833585). For parents of children born with heart disease. Includes a bereavement group. Groups and contacts mainly in the North of England. (See also Heartline Association.)

**Association for Spina Bifida and Hydrocephalus (ASBAH)**

ASBAH House, 42 Park Road, Peterborough PE1 2UQ (0733 555988). For parents of children with neural tube defects.

**British Diabetic Association**

10 Queen Anne Street, London W1M 0BD (071 323 1531). For people with diabetes.

**British Epilepsy Association**

Anstey house, 40 Hanover Square, Leeds LS3 1BE (information: 0532 439393/helpline: 0345 089599). For people with epilepsy.

**Epilepsy Associaton of Scotland**

48 Govan Road, Glasgow G51 1JL (041 427 4911).

**British Epilepsy Association Northern Ireland Region**

The Old Postgraduate Medical Centre, Belfast City Hospital, Lisburn Road, Belfast BT9 7AB (0232 248 414).

**British Heart Foundation**

4 Fitzhardinge Street, London W1H 4DH (071 935 0185). For people with heart disease and for parents of children born with heart problems.

**British Kidney Patients Association**

Bordon, Hampshire GU35 9JZ (0420 472021). For people with kidney disease.

**Cervical Stitch Network**

Fairfield, Wolverton Road, Norton Lindsey, Warwick CV35 8LA. For women who have or are considering having a cervical stitch in pregnancy; part of the Miscarriage Association (see above).

**Contact-A-Family**

16 Strutton Ground, London SW1P 2HP (071 222 2695). For parents of children born with disabilities and handicapping conditions. Links with local and national groups.

**Cytomegalovirus Support Group**

69 The Leasowes, Ford, Shrewsbury, Shropshire SY5 9LU (0743 850055). For parents whose babies have been damaged by cytomegalovirus (CMV).

**Diabetes Foundation**

177a Tennison Road, London SE25 5NF(24 hour helpline: 081 656 5467). For people with diabetes.

**Down's Syndrome Association**

155 Mitcham Road, Tooting, London SW17 9PG (081 682 4001). For parents of children born with Down's syndrome.

**Heartline Association**
12 Cremer Place, The Chestnuts, Wildish Road, Faversham. Kent ME13 7SG (0795 539864). For parents of children born with heart disease. Includes a bereavement group. Groups and contacts mainly in the south and east of England. (See also Association of Children with Heart Disorders).

**Herpes Association**
41 North Road, London N7 9DP (071 609 9061). For people with herpes.

**In Touch**
10 Norman Road, Sale, Cheshire M33 3DF (061 905 2440). Provides individual links with parents of children born with rare medical conditions.

**Lupus UK**
Queens Court, 9 – 17 Eastern Road, Romford, Essex RM1 3NG (0708 731251). For people with lupus (systematic lupus erythematosus or SLE). There is also a lupus adviser in the Welfare Department of Arthritis Care, 6 Grosvenor Crescent, London SW1X 7ER (071 235 0902/3/4/5).

**Potter's Syndrome Support Group**
46 Borfa-Green, Welshpool, Powys SY21 7QF (0938 553755). For parents of children born with Potter's syndrome.

**Pre-Eclamptic Toxaemia Society (PETS)**
Eaton Lodge, 8 Southend Road, Hockley, Essex SS5 4QQ (0702 205088). For people who suffer from pregnancy-induced hypertension (pre-eclampsia or pre-eclamptic toxaemia).

**Rare Unspecified Chromosome Disorder Support Group**
160 Locket Road, Harrow Weald, Middx HA3 7NZ (081 863 3557). For parents of children born with a rare unspecified chromosome disorder.

**Sense – The National Deaf-Blind and Rubella Organisation**
311 Grays Inn Road, London WC1X 8PT (071 278 1005). For information about rubella and for parents of children affected by rubella.

**Sickle Cell Society**
54 Station Road, Harlesden, London NW10 7VA (081 961 7795). For people with sickle cell disease or sickle cell trait. Can refer to genetic counselling centres.

**SOFT UK (Support Organisation for Trisomy 13/18 and related disorders)**
National Co-ordinator Trisomy 13 (Patau's syndrome), Tudor Lodge, Redwood, Ross-on-Wye, Herefordshire HR9 5UD (0989 67480). National Co-ordinator Trisomy 18 (Edwards' syndrome), 48 Froggatt's Ride, Walmley, Sutton Coldfield, West Midlands B76 8TQ (021 351 3122). For parents of children born with Trisomy 13 (Patau's syndrome), Trisomy 18 (Edwards' syndrome) or related chromosomal disorders.

**Toxoplasmosis Trust**
Room 26, 61 – 71 Collier Street, London N1 0BE (071 713 0599). For information about toxoplasmosis and support for people who have had it.

**Turner's Syndrome Society**
2 Mayfield Avenue, Chiswick, London W4 1PW (081 994 7625). For parents of children with Turner's syndrome.

**UK Thalassaemia Society**
107 Nightingale Lane, London N8 7QY (081 348 0437). For people with
thalassaemia, carriers and their families.


## MORE GENERAL COUNSELLING, ADVICE AND SUPPORT

**Action for Victims of Medical Accidents (AVMA)**
Bank Chambers, 1 London Road, Forest Hill, London SE23 3TP (081 291
2793). Works for the fair treatment of victims of medical accidents. Advice
and support.

**Association of Community Health Councils for England and Wales (ACHCEW)**
30 Drayton Park, London N5 1PB (071 609 8405). Community Health
Councils (Local Health Councils in Scotland, Area Health Councils in
Northern Ireland) are independent watchdogs over local health services
and can support people who wish to complain about the care they or
members of their family have received. For the address and telephone
number of the local Community Health Council or equivalent, see the
local phone book or contact the relevant association.

**Association of Scottish Local Health Councils**
21 Torpichen Street, Edinburgh EH3 8 HX (031 229 2344).

**Association of Area Health Councils**
c/o Central Services Agency, 25–7 Adelaide Street, Belfast BT2 8FH
(0232 324431).

**British Association for Counselling**
37a Sheep Street, Rugby, Warwickshire CV21 3BX (0788 578328/9).
Information on where to get counselling locally.

**Catholic Marriage Advisory Council**
Clitherow House, 1 Blythe Mews, Blythe Road, London W14 0NW (071
371 1341). Marriage and relationship counselling.

**Compassionate Friends**
6 Denmark Street, Bristol BS1 5DQ (0272 292778). Support for parents
of children who have died.

**CRUSE – Bereavement Care**
Cruse House, 126 Sheen Road, Richmond, Surrey TW9 1UR (081 940
4818). Support and advice for the bereaved.

**Jewish Bereavement Counselling Service**
1 Cyprus Gardens, London N3 1SP (071 387 4300 x227/24 hour
answerphone: 081 349 0839). Bereavement counselling.

**London Bereavement Projects Co-ordinating Group**
c/o 68 Chalton Street, London NW1 1JR (24 hour answerphone: 071 388
2153). Counselling and support for anyone who is bereaved. Referral to a
local bereavement project.

**NAFSIYAT**
278 Seven Sisters Road, London N4 2HY (071 263 4130). Short-term counselling and psychotherapy for Black and ethnic minorities.

**RELATE**
Herbert Gray College, Little Church Street, Rugby, Warwickshire CV21 3AP (0788 573241; or see under Relate in the local telephone book). Confidential counselling for relationship problems of any kind.

**Samaritans**
17 Uxbridge Road, Slough, Berks SL1 1SN (0753 32713/4; or see under Samaritans in the local telephone book). 24 hour confidential telephone help for people who are in despair, some of whom feel suicidal.

**Westminster Pastoral Foundation**
23 Kensington Square, London W8 5HN (071 937 6956). Individual, marital and family counselling. Information on similar services in other parts of the UK.

## PREGNANCY, CHILDBIRTH AND GENERAL

**Active Birth Centre**
55 Dartmouth Park Road, London NW5 1SL (071 267 3006). Information and advice on active birth.

**Alcohol Concern**
305 Gray's Inn Road, London WC1X 8QF (071 833 3471). Advice and information about sensible drinking. Addresses of local alcohol advisory agencies.

**Scottish Council on Alcohol**
137 – 45 Sauchiehall Street, Glasgow G2 3EW(041 333 9677).

**Northern Ireland Council on Alcohol**
40 Elmwood Avenue, Belfast BT9 6AZ (0232 664 434).

**Association for Improvements in the Maternity Services (AIMS)**
21 Iver Lane, Iver, Bucks SLO 9LH (0753 652781). Advice on rights, complaints procedures and choices in maternity care.

**Association for Post-Natal Illness**
25 Jerdan Place, London SW6 1BE (10a.m.–12p.m. 071 386 0868). Support and advice from other mothers who have recovered from post-natal illness.

**British Agencies for Adoption and Fostering (BAAF)**
11 Southwark Street, London SE1 1RQ (071 407 8800). Offers advice and information to people considering adoption and fostering.

**Caesarean Support Network**
2 Hurst Park Drive, Huyton, Liverpool L36 1TF (051 480 1184). Friendly non-medical advice about caesarean sections.

**CHILD**
PO Box 154, Hounslow TW3 0EZ (081 571 4376). Support and information for families with infertility problems.

**Family Planning Information Service (FPIS)**
27 – 35 Mortimer Street, London W1N 7RJ (071 636 7866). Information

on infertility and sexual difficulties. Referral to local sources of help.

**Foresight**

The Old Vicarage, Church Lane, Witley, Goldalming, Surrey GU8 5PN (0428 684500). Aims to improve couples' health before pregnancy.

**Issue – National Fertility Association**

St George's Rectory, Tower Street, Birmingham B19 3UY (021 359 4887). Advice and information for people with infertility and related problems.

**Maternity Alliance**

15 Britannia Street, London WC1X 9JP (071 837 1265). Information on maternity care and rights.

**National Childbirth Trust (NCT)**

Alexandra House, Oldham Terrace, Acton, London W3 6NH (081 992 8637). Advice and information on pregnancy and childbirth. Local support groups and classes. Local contacts for parents who have lost a baby. Also has a contact register for parents with disabilities and chronic disease.

**QUIT**

Latimer House, 102 Gloucester Place, London W1H 3DA (071 487 3000 – Smokers' Quitline). Information and advice for people who want to give up smoking. Addresses of local support groups.

## AUSTRALIA

The Department of Health in each state produces brochures on maternal and perinatal care. Social workers of major maternity hospitals will generally have information on support groups and other useful addresses.

**Compassionate Friends**

Bereaved Parents Support and Information Centre, Lower Parish Hall, 300 Camberwell Road, Camberwell, Vic 3124 (03 882 3355).

**Family Planning Federation of Australia**

Suite 3, 1st Floor, LUA Building, 39 Geils Court, Deakin, ACT 2600 (062 85 1244). Provides counselling and an advice and referral service for women. Contact for local branch.

**Maternity Alliance**

PO Box 314, Katoomba, NSW 2780 (02 477 1464).

**National Association of Loss and Grief**

Qld, NSW, Vic.

Please contact your state office, listed in relevent telephone directory.

**SELAG (South Australian Association of Loss and Grief)**

Listed in relevent telephone directory.

**WELAG (Western Australian Association of Loss and Grief)**

Listed in relevant telephone directory.

**Stillbirth and Neonatal Death Support (SANDS)**

(ACT) PO Box 204, Curtin, ACT 2605 (06 258 7569/292 4330).

(NSW) Level 3/Block 4, Royal North Shore Hospital, Pacific Highway,

St Leonards, NSW 2065 (02 906 7004).
(Qld) PO Box 708, South Brisbane, Qld 4101 (07 207 1397).
(SA) PO Box 380, Parkholme, SA 5043 (08 277 0304).
(Tas) PO Box 874, Devonport, Tas 7310 (004 26 1137).
(Vic) 19 Canterbury Road, Camberwell, Vic 3124 (03 882 1590).
(WA) Agnes Walsh House, King Edward Memorial Hospital, Bagot Road, Subiaco, WA 6008 (09 382 2687).

## NEW ZEALAND

**Compassionate Friends NZ**
Ms Patsy Holly, 9 Welles Street, Ranfurly, Otago, or Ms Nina Sandilands, 16 Parkes Avenue, Wanganui.
**NZ Family Planning Association**
National Office, PO Box 11515, Wellington (04 844 349).
**Pregnancy Help**
National Office, PO Box 12 – 000, Wellington.
**Stillbirth and Neonatal Death (SANDS)**
30 Church Street, Palmerston North.

## USA

**Boston Women's Health Collective**
240a Elm Street, Sommerville, MA 02144. Women's health information centre.
**Compassionate Friends**
PO Box 3696, Oak Brook, Ill 60522 – 3696 (708 990 0100).
Organisation offering support to bereaved parents and siblings.
**Elizabeth Kubler-Ross Center**
South Route, 616, Head Waters, Va 24442 (703 396 3441). A non-profit, non- sectarian organisation dedicated to the enhancement of people's lives. There are support groups in most states.
**Good Grief Program**
Judge Baker Children's Center, 295 Longwood Avenue, Boston, MA 02155.
**ICEA (International Childbirth Education Association)**
PO Box 20048, Minneapolis, Minnesota 55420 (612 854 8660).
**Life Center of the Suncoats Inc**
214 S. Fielding Avenue, Tampa, FL 33606 (813 251 0289). Offers support to people experiencing the stresses of serious illness or loss.
**National Commission to Prevent Infant Mortality**
Switzer Building, Rm 2014, 330 C Street SW, Washington, DC 20201 (202 472 1364).
**Pregnancy and Infant Loss Center**
Tel: 612 473 9372. For bereaved families who have experienced miscarriage, stillbirth and infant death.

**SIDS (Sudden Infant Death Syndrome Alliance)**
10500 Little Patuxent Parkway, Suite 420, Columbia, Maryland 21044
(800 221 7437/410 964 8000).

# Index

| | | | |
|---|---|---|---|
| 0 04 440 4913 | *Miscarriage* Christine Moulder | £5.99 | ☐ |
| 0 04 440 5669 | *When a Baby Dies* Nancy Kohner & Alix Henley | £6.99 | ☐ |
| 0 04 440 7386 | *The Caesarean Experience* Sarah Clement | £6.99 | ☐ |
| 0 04 440 08455 | *The Midwife Challenge* Ed. Sheila Kitzinger | £6.99 | ☐ |
| 0 8635 80475 | *Birth and Our Bodies* Paddy O'Brien | £5.99 | ☐ |

All these books are available at your local bookseller or can be ordered direct from the publishers.

To order direct just tick the titles you want and fill in the form below:

Name: _____

Address: _____

_____

_____ Post Code: _____

Send to: Thorsons Mail Order, Dept 31G, HarperCollins*Publishers*, Westerhill Road, Bishopbriggs, Glasgow G64 2QT.

Please enclose a cheque or postal order or debit my Visa/Access account —

Credit card no: _____

Expiry date: _____

Signature: _____

— to the value of the cover price plus:

**UK & BFPO:** Add £1.00 for the first book and 25p for each additional book ordered.

**Overseas orders including Eire:** Please add £2.95 service charge. Books will be sent by surface mail but quotes for airmail despatches will be given on request.

**24 HOUR TELEPHONE ORDERING SERVICE** FOR ACCESS/ VISA CARDHOLDERS — TEL: **041 772 2281.**